T0116434

LivClear
and Thrive
DETOXIFICATION PROGRAM

A Personal Guide To A Bio-Transformational
and Life Changing Experience

Dr. Christopher Bump

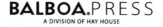

BALBOA.PRESS
A DIVISION OF HAY HOUSE

Balboa Press books may be ordered through booksellers or by contacting:

Balboa Press
A Division of Hay House
1663 Liberty Drive
Bloomington, IN 47403
www.balboapress.com
844-682-1282

Print information available on the last page.

ISBN: 979-8-7652-4727-3 (sc)
ISBN: 979-8-7652-4729-7 (hc)
ISBN: 979-8-7652-4728-0 (e)

Library of Congress Control Number: 2023922412

Balboa Press rev. date: 12/15/2023

CONTENTS

Part III Dr. Bump's Recipes

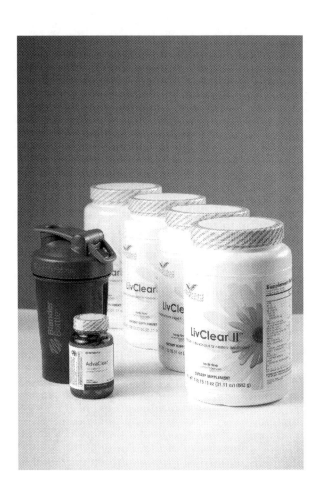

INTRODUCTION

Congratulations on choosing to be an active participant in your health. During the next four weeks, you'll be creating a solid foundation for lifestyle changes that can provide health-enhancing improvements for the rest of your life. And I don't say that lightly.

Although the idea of detoxification may seem daunting, you will soon discover through this easy-to-follow program that feeling healthy is just a few changes away. And you may be surprised to see these positive changes affecting many different aspects of your life.

When discussing health, one must include the mind, body, and spirit—all of which will be addressed during this program. Now, let's get into the good stuff!

Why Detox Anyway?

The idea of detoxification has been around for centuries. Consequently, all kinds of therapies and protocols have been devised to detoxify our bodies. Toxins are defined as any substance either taken in from the environment or created within our own bodies that does not serve a useful physiologic function and typically damages our health.

Herbs, bowel cleansing, fasts, steams, and saunas are a few of the ways our ancestors detoxed. And over eons we have developed a very elaborate system, consisting mostly of liver enzymes, to break down and clean out toxic debris. In the past, the toxic waste we needed to remove came mostly from plants and microbes, along with our own cellular garbage.

We need to keep our bodies free of toxins, as research has clearly established the accumulation of toxins as a major contributor to poor health. Toxins come from all kinds of sources in the environment, such as water, air, soil, and food. Given the current condition of our Great Mother Earth, it is clear we are exposed to thousands of toxins every day. In fact, it is estimated that we are subjected to over 50,000 manufacture chemicals and over 1,500 organophosphates in our environment (I call these "new-to-nature" substances). In 2019, according to the U.S. Environmental

Protection Agency, over three billion pounds of chemical pollutants were released into the environment. Toxins can be derived from:

- Chemical pollutants
- Industrial manufacturing
- Heavy metals
- Drugs
- Pesticides
- Herbicides
- Food additives
- Cigarette smoke (either passive or active)
- Alcohol
- Home care products
- Cosmetics

Additionally, toxins come from an intestinal buildup of unhealthy flora, viral overload such as from Epstein Bar Virus and normal metabolic activity, as mentioned above. Over the span of our lives, we come into contact with more toxins than we can detoxify. Most food, water and air is riddled with toxicants. So, no one escapes being exposed to the environmental burden of "new to nature" chemicals. This may be sad to think of, but there is hope— it's what the LivClear Detox Program is all about!

How each person will be affected by a detoxification program is really up to the individual. Each of us is unique—not just our specific personalities, but also our own biochemistry. Just as no two snowflakes are alike, the same is true for humans. However, everyone who participates in the LivClear Detox Program will benefit, because for the most part, we all have the same detoxing capabilities. And most will have positive, clear, and obvious results with the four-week program. You may struggle for a short time with cravings, slight body aches, or headaches, but these clearing symptoms are short-lived and will soon be behind you. As Brendon Bouchard says, "Honor the struggle!" Here are some of the benefits typically experienced:

- Increased energy
- Balanced hormones
- Weight loss

- Improved neurologic function
- Better sleep
- Fewer aches and pains
- Decreased cravings
- Stronger immunity
- Clearer thinking
- Improved digestion
- Reduced muscle tension
- Reduced oxidative stress
- Healthier bowel movements
- Decreased headache and migraine
- Better attitude
- Greater enjoyment of food
- Greater productivity
- Enhanced social responsibility

I am often asked if people with specific conditions and "diseases" will benefit from doing the LivClear Detox Program. And it is important for you to know that this program does NOT treat diseases. However, when you begin to understand that what we call diseases are really a compilation of imbalances in your organs and glands, then getting to the root cause may have an effect on the symptoms associated with a "disease." I can safely say that there are a host of conditions that have shown improvement with the LivClear Detox Program. Some of them include the following, but the list is not exclusive:

- Fibromyalgia
- Osteo and rheumatoid arthritis
- Chronic fatigue syndrome
- Elevated cholesterol
- Hypertension (increased blood pressure)
- Diabetes
- Hypoglycemia
- Eczema and psoriasis
- Allergy
- Asthma

- Hormone imbalances like PMS
- Chemical sensitivity
- Insomnia
- Chronic inflammation
- Autoimmune conditions
- Irritable bowel syndrome (IBS), gastro-esophageal reflux disease (GERD), indigestion

How Our Body Detoxes

The term "detoxification" refers to our body's natural ability to transform, transfer, and eliminate toxins. As medical science has evolved, so has our understanding of how our bodies process toxins. We have gained a fairly clear picture of the nutritional biochemistry involved in breaking down and eliminating these substances.

The detoxification process of transforming toxicants mostly involves the liver. The kidneys, skin, lungs, gall bladder/biliary system, and intestines also help. The immune system (comprised of white blood cells), the circulatory system (comprised of the vascular system), the lymphatic system, and adipose tissue all help to move and store toxins as well.

A substance must be able to dissolve in water for it to be easily eliminated from the body. This is why we have to detoxify toxicants in the first place, since toxins simply don't dissolve out of your body easily on their own. Typically, most toxic compounds are manufactured and stored as fatty molecules and therefore do not mix well with water. Think of oil and water. The detoxification process transforms these fatty, oil-like agents to water-soluble molecules, which can then be excreted from the body.

The detoxification process can be summarized in three phases:

Phase One: Liver function (part one), also known as the cytochrome P-450 pathways:

- Fat-soluble toxins are transformed into intermediate compounds, which are very reactive and hence more toxic. These join more easily to nontoxic, antioxidant, water-soluble molecules in Phase Two.

Phase Two: Liver function (part two), also known as the conjugation pathways:

- Joining of the newly formed reactive intermediate molecules with water-soluble nutrients make the entire compound harmless and easier to excrete from the body.
- Without enough nutrient support of the Phase Two process, the highly reactive intermediates can damage healthy tissues and may lead to pathology. These toxicants create free radicals and increase oxidative stress, which further damages our cells. This is the primary reason for elevated cholesterol and most chronic inflammatory illness.

Phase Three: Excretion

- Neutralized toxins, now made water-soluble, are removed from the body in the urine via the kidneys, or the bile/feces through the intestinal tract.

Think of the detoxification process like a septic system you find in rural homes. The effluent travels out through our drainpipes to the septic tank, where bacteria work on reducing the waste to small particulate compounds. The intermediate form of waste is then leached out into the earth, where it is further reduced to organic compounds by microbes in the soil. It then becomes nontoxic and recycles with the soil—hopefully!

What About Fasting?

It should become obvious that fasting, either with just water or juices, may not be the best thing for our detoxification process. While fasting has been used for centuries in both physical and spiritual practices, it is not a recommended practice any longer, mostly because of the toxic chemical burden we place on our body as modern humans.

Many years ago, before synthetic (think new-to-nature) chemicals were introduced into our lives, fasting was a viable way to help our ancestors survive long and cold winters. When food became scarce, fasting was a natural way to consume less. Also, most cultures fasted as a spiritual practice to control the attachment to earthly pleasures.

Today, given the levels of chemical toxins we are subject to and the levels of stress under which we live, fasting is not a healthy or recommended option. You may have heard a newer term lately that has become quite popular, called intermittent fasting. This is a viable option for some, once they are out of insulin resistance and metabolic syndrome. However, detoxifying your body first, before beginning the practice of intermittent fasting, is highly advised and recommended.

As you will learn, there is a significant amount of nutritional biochemistry involved in the detoxification process. These biochemical pathways need to be fortified and supported continually, but during your LivClear Detoxification Program they will need even more fortification and support.

Nutrients Required For Detox Support

The nutrients required for supporting the three phases of your detox are extensive. Some of them may sound familiar, but many are complex molecules that are best consumed in supplement form. The LivClear II detoxification shake provides all the necessary nutrients to break fat-soluble toxins into water-soluble intermediates. To emphasize, the LivClear II formula is not doing the detoxifying. That's your liver's job! It simply provides the nutrient ingredients to best support the liver during the detoxification process. Some of those nutrients are:

- Vitamins A, B3, B6, B12, C, and E
- Beta-carotene
- Folate
- Amino acids such as L-cysteine, L-glutamine, and taurine
- Zinc
- Pantothenic acid
- N-acetyecysteine
- Sodium sulphate
- Glutathione
- Green tea catechin

During the LivClear Program, all of these nutrients are provided in a palatable medicinal food drink that will be consumed throughout the 28-day program. Were you worried you'd have to take a ton of pills each day? Using this medicinal food shake makes it unnecessary to take handfuls of supplements. Through many years of offering this program to thousands of individuals just like you, I have found that this meal replacement shake is a great tool for change. It also creates an opportunity for much greater compliance than taking pills.

How Will Detoxification Make Me Feel?

Since each of us has our own unique biochemistry, state of health, and history, every person will respond to the LivClear Detox Program differently. We've found 99 percent of individuals who have gone through the program have had significant positive results.

Deliberately changing your lifestyle is a positive step toward living a healthier life. When you choose to stop consuming sugar, alcohol, and wheat, you will go through a period of withdrawal both mentally and physically. Sugar, alcohol, wheat, and dairy are addictive, and they increase your dopamine levels and endorphins. These foods also have a negative effect on your blood sugar levels and your immune system. Some individuals experience minimal reactions and others have only mild withdrawal symptoms of irritability, headache, and lethargy for a day or two. And some have a more intense reaction that can take a week or two to overcome.

As you can imagine, the reactions are different in everyone depending on many variables. But I want to reassure you that in the many years I have prescribed this program, very few have not been able to overcome the reactions they have experienced. The fact that you are choosing to take care of yourself is a positive step, so continually remind yourself of all the benefits you will derive from going through the LivClear Detoxification Program.

PROGRAM OVERVIEW

Every BODY is different. The LivClear Detox Program is 28 days, but it can be adjusted to meet the requirements of each person. Over the course of the program, you will be drinking the LivClear II medicinal food, which can be a meal replacement at the full dose of two scoops per shake. You will slowly increase the amount of LivClear you're consuming each day and adjust the amount of food you eat to satisfy your hunger. This is an important rule that will be repeated often. **You should never ignore your hunger.**

Also, one of the reasons this program was created to be 28 days, is that research shows you have to repeat a new behavior every day for 21 days for it to become a regular part of your life or what's better known as . . . a good habit!

You will start the LivClear Program by drinking the beverage in small amounts. That's so you do not overload your detoxification pathways too quickly. You will slowly increase the number of shakes each day and eventually reach a dose where you won't be eating solid foods. By the end of Day 7, you will be drinking enough LivClear II to satisfy your metabolic and nutritional needs. At this stage of the program, listening to your body is critical for determining whether or not your eating schedule needs to be adjusted. Use your appetite as a barometer. It's important to note that individuals who are insulin resistant, in metabolic syndrome, or used to high carbohydrate diets may take a week or two to shift their metabolism. Remember the rule—**never ignore your hunger!**

Days 7–11 are when you will have LivClear II only, and that's often when the greatest benefits are experienced. Going five days without solid food allows the body to begin to recuperate from the many years of being overburdened every single day. On Day 12, you will begin to reduce the number of LivClear II shakes and start to reintroduce foods from the Basic Dietary Guidelines. There's no need to worry about which foods to enjoy, as each day of the LivClear Detox Program is outlined in detail with plenty of suggestions and advice to make the whole process easy.

You will consume four containers of LivClear II during 28 days. However, some individuals begin feeling so good during the process that they extend the no-food portion of the program. The longest time thus far has been three months! Yes, this means you can live on the LivClear shake.

The Basic Dietary Guidelines (listed below) are based on an elimination diet that is used to remove food allergens and toxic substances (although I find it difficult to call chemicalized substances food). These are foods that are known to cause some immune reaction in almost everyone, so they are eliminated during the program.

Let me explain an important point about the Basic Dietary Guidelines you will be following. Close to 80 percent of your body's immune system works in and around the intestinal tract. It is the first line of defense against the microbial pathogens, environmental toxins, and chemicals you take in. These are found in the food you eat, water you drink, and drugs you may take. The immune system is there to protect you! Help it function at its best by removing substances that continually stimulate it into action. By removing known antigenic foods and eating organic and chemical-free food, your immune system can take a much-needed break.

BASIC DIETARY GUIDELINES

Fruits:

- *INCLUDE:* Unsweetened fresh, water-packed, or canned fruits. Organic when possible.
- *OMIT:* All fruit juices. Bananas (eliminate all uses). Oranges, including orange juice. Oranges are a high-allergen food, and orange juice is loaded with aspergillus yeast.

Vegetables:

- *INCLUDE:* All fresh, raw, steamed, sautéed, juiced, or roasted vegetables. Sweet potatoes are allowed. Organic when possible.
- *OMIT:* Creamed vegetables. White potatoes.

Starch (bread/cereal): Keep this category to a minimum or completely omit.

- *INCLUDE:* Rice, oats, millet, quinoa, amaranth, teff, tapioca, buckwheat, and related products. This can include pasta, bread, crackers, flours, etc. Organic and whole when possible.
- *OMIT:* Wheat, corn, rye, barley, spelt, kamut, and any gluten-containing product. If weight loss is a goal, then keep this category of foods either minimal or eliminate completely.
  * Gluten (the allergen protein found in wheat, pasta, bagels, pancakes, etc.) is the most "antigenic" protein and causes an amazing array of health conditions. Most gluten-free products are made from potatoes, which are not allowed.
- Oats are often processed in the same facilities as wheat and therefore are cross contaminated with gluten. Also, oats do not have gluten but a different group of proteins called avenins.
- All grains are high in starchy carbohydrates, which increase blood sugar and insulin.

Legumes (vegetable proteins):

- *INCLUDE:* All beans, peas, and lentils. Organic when possible.
- *OMIT:* Soybeans, tofu, tempeh, soy milk, and other soy products. *Soy in limited amounts and in certain forms is acceptable after the detox program. Soy is a highly allergenic food protein.

Nuts and Seeds:

- *INCLUDE:* Almonds, walnuts, sesame (tahini), sunflower, and pumpkin seeds. Butters made from these nuts and seeds. Organic when possible.
- *OMIT:* Cashews, peanuts, and peanut butters. Peanuts tend to be a very moldy nut and are loaded with aflatoxins (aka fungus poop!).

Meat and Fish (animal protein):

- *INCLUDE:* All canned (water-packed), frozen, or fresh fish, chicken, turkey, wild game, and lamb. Free-range and organically fed when possible. Grass-fed beef and pork are encouraged.
- *OMIT:* Commercially raised beef, pork, eggs, shellfish, cold cuts, frankfurters, sausage, and canned meats.
  *Meats are loaded with growth-enhancing drugs and antibiotics. They also contain a high percentage of saturated and trans fats.

Dairy Products and Milk Substitutes:

- *INCLUDE:* Milk substitutes such as almond milk, hemp milk, macadamia milk, and coconut milk.
- *OMIT:* Milk, cheese, cottage cheese, cream, ice cream, yogurt, butter, and nondairy creamers.
  *Casein is the allergenic protein in all dairy products. It is hard on our immunity and our intestinal tract. It also makes lots of mucous.

Fats:

- *INCLUDE:* Cold-pressed olive, canola, sesame, safflower, sunflower, walnut, hemp, pumpkin, and almond oils. Ghee, which is clarified butter, is encouraged.
- *OMIT:* Margarine, butter, shortening, partially hydrogenated and hydrogenated oils, mayonnaise, spreads, cotton seed, and soy oils. *Fats and oils cause significant oxidative damage to our cellular membranes.

Beverages:

- *INCLUDE:* Filtered or distilled water, herbal teas, naturally carbonated or mineral waters. Green tea may be used to wean off of coffee; keep to a minimum.
- *OMIT:* Soda and soft drinks, alcoholic beverages, coffee, black tea, and other caffeinated beverages.

Spices and Condiments:

- *INCLUDE* All spices unless otherwise noted. For example, carob, cinnamon, cumin, dill, garlic, ginger, oregano, parsley, rosemary, tarragon, thyme, turmeric, and vinegar. Organic is recommended because spices and herbs are concentrated and contain pesticides and herbicides if commercially produced.
- *OMIT:* Chocolate, ketchup, mustard, relish, chutney, soy sauce, barbecue sauce, and other condiments.

Sweeteners: Minimal to none

- *INCLUDE:* Brown rice syrup, fruit sweeteners, and blackstrap molasses.
- *OMIT:* Sugar (white or brown), honey, maple syrup, stevia, corn syrup, high fructose corn syrup, candy, and desserts, etc.

GUIDES, REMINDERS, AND WARNINGS

Suggested LivClear II mixing instructions:

- Due to settling of the powder, shake the container several times before opening. Using the scoop provided, mix the amount of LivClear II recommended in your program with 8 to 10 ounces of water or other liquid, such as hemp, macadamia, or almond milk or coconut drink (not coconut water). Add ice if desired. Use a shaker mug or blender until well mixed, and then drink slowly. Think of it as food!
- You may use LivClear II as part of your meal or as a meal replacement. It can also be blended with a variety of fruits (if allowed) and other liquids as mentioned above. Remember, if you are interested in weight reduction, adding fruit and "milks" adds calories as well. A serving of LivClear II mixed in water is approximately 165 calories.
- For the first three days, it is suggested to use only water for mixing LivClear II. This provides an opportunity to discover both its taste and texture.
- After Day 3, you may begin using either unsweetened almond, hemp, or macadamia milk, or blended fresh fruit if allowed. Berries are best! Mix 1:1 less or more according to taste and caloric need. For example, someone with a high, fast metabolism will need extra calories throughout the program.

Mixing Variations:

For all the recipes below, mix the ingredients in a blender (if using whole pieces of fruit) or a shaker cup. Add 8 to 10 ounces of water, or desired liquid, and blend or shake to desired consistency. Adjust liquid according to personal taste.

- 6 to 8 ounces of water, 2 or 3 ice cubes, and one of the following: ½ apple or peach, 1 or 2 slices pineapple, or ¼ to ½ cup berries.

- 3 to 4 ounces of water, 3 to 4 ounces allowable milk substitutes, 2 or 3 ice cubes, and fresh fruit as above.
- 6 to 8 ounces allowable milk substitute (plain), and 2 to 3 ice cubes or frozen fruit (berries, peaches, or apples).

Side Note: Adding other vegetable and nut milks makes the LivClear II shake smoother, sweeter, and tastier. It also, however, adds approximately 120 calories per 8 fluid ounces depending on the mix. Please remember and respect this rule, as keeping your blood sugar stable is extremely important.

Water Intake:

- How much water should you drink every day? Take your weight, divide that number in half, and drink that many ounces of water per day. For example, if you weigh 140 pounds, half of that is 70 ounces of water per day.
- Water should be clean, filtered, bottled, or otherwise uncontaminated.

Activity Levels:

- Rest is important, so eight hours of sleep each night is ideal. If possible, try and rest (nap) for a half hour to an hour each day, especially during the five days of consuming only LivClear II.
- Regardless of your exercise routine, slow it down from your usual pace and intensity. Go easy. Exercise very lightly. This can include walks, gentle yoga, stationary bike, and treadmill. Do not lift weights or engage in vigorous workouts from Days 6 to 16.
- Avoid STRESS as much as possible and find time each day for quiet and relaxation.

Possible Side Effects, Reactions and Symptoms:

You might experience sensations and symptoms that are not pleasant during the first week of the detox program. But please don't be alarmed by this as some are expected and indicate cellular and organ change. These can be:

- Headache

- Increased body aches
- Fatigue
- Sleep disturbances
- Gastrointestinal symptoms

During the five days with no food, if you experience any signs or symptoms of lightheadedness, severe hunger, fatigue, or anything related to low blood sugar, eat allowable foods in the basic dietary guidelines.

Sluggish Bowels:

The LivClear Detox Program will change many things for you in several positive ways. Because you will be going through significant dietary changes, and consuming the LivClear II in increasing amounts, you might experience changes in your bowel habits. Don't be alarmed about this, as it is the result of a shift in your microbiome and how you utilize your water. I can honestly say I have never had anyone experience diarrhea, or "disaster pants," as Dave Asprey of Bulletproof fame likes to say. If you have any negative reaction at all, experiencing a slowing down of your bowels is much more likely. But there is an easy, safe, and beneficial way to promote healthy bowels should they slow down. Here's what to do.

Magnesium Citrate Loading:

Purchase pure magnesium citrate from a reputable manufacturer of nutrient supplements. The dose per capsule should be 125 mg.

- Begin with two capsules or about 250 mg, with food or shake. Magnesium can cause a bit of nausea if taken on an empty stomach.
- Take another two capsules every three to four hours until you have a bowel movement. It is probable that your stool will be quite loose or even diarrhea.
- Keep track of how many doses it takes for your bowels to wake up. This will give you an idea of how deficient in magnesium you are and how much you'll need to take every day to keep things moving.
- You'll want to find your own "sweet spot" for how much you'll need on a daily basis.

Continue your required dosage on a daily basis, and usually the amount you need will diminish within a few days or weeks. But do continue with the magnesium as it has many more benefits than just hydrating your colon.

- It is essential for energy, muscle relaxation, protein production, nerve transmission, calming, and about three hundred other biochemical processes.
- Similarly, you can use vitamin C to hydrate your colon and your stool, though the dosing is quite different. I'd recommend using magnesium first and go to the vitamin C as a second option.
- Use pure buffered ascorbic acid and begin with 2000 mg. Increase the dose by 1000 mg every six to eight hours. Again, keep track of how much vitamin C it takes to get you moving, and reduce by 25 percent the next day.
- Using vitamin C loading offers incredible antioxidant benefits as well.

Warnings and Disclaimers

This program is intended to provide information to create a change in lifestyle, not to treat any specific medical condition. It is therefore not intended as a substitute for treatment, diagnostics, or any health care services. If you suspect you have a medical condition or any health-related matter, please consult a competent medical practitioner, preferably one who is certified by the Institute for Functional Medicine (IFM.org)

As you go through the LivClear Detoxification Program, it is probable that you will have some degree of discomfort in a few areas. I will list the most common types of reactions, their causes, and remedies.

Caffeine withdrawal headache: This is the most common adverse reaction I see. Anyone who has enjoyed coffee habitually, will probably experience a headache. The most common cause is due to caffeine's vasoconstriction effect. When you omit caffeine cold turkey, your blood vessels, which are used to the constriction, dilate, increasing blood flow and pressure in your head.

Remedy: Wait it out, as it usually lasts no more than a day. Drink lots of water, and if needed, take an over-the-counter pain med. If taking an Advil, Tylenol, or aspirin will keep you in the driver's seat, then do so.

Hunger: If you have blood-sugar-handling issues like hypoglycemia, if you are pre-diabetic, insulin resistant, or overweight, or if you have slightly elevated hemoglobin A1C and blood glucose, then it will take you a week to ten days to shift your metabolism. This is extremely important to remember, because when your body is used to using sugars, starches, and carbohydrates for fuel, and you remove them, your brain will be going into "hunt" mode!

Remedy: *Do not ignore your hunger. Eat within 10 to 15 minutes!* You must have either a shake or food from the program. Clean-sourced meat and fat is best. You can also add some quality fat to your shake, like ghee, coconut oil or Medium Chain Triglycerides (MCT) oil, or you can have a clean-sourced protein powder.

Drowsiness and Fatigue: Your metabolism is going to change and will begin to process and utilize nutrients much more efficiently. However, it takes a few days to a week or more to push your cells this way, so during this transition time, you may experience fluctuations in blood sugar levels which can cause you to feel tired.

Remedy: See the rule above under Hunger. Increase your protein intake throughout the day. Add a scoop of a quality protein powder to the LivClear II shake, like clean-sourced whey proteins such as Metagenics BioPure Protein.

Irritability: You may find yourself a bit more irritable than usual in the first 5 to 7 days of the program. There are several reasons for this, with the first related to the issue discussed above—fluctuations in blood sugar. Hypoglycemia (low blood sugar) will cause irritability, usually in the afternoon or evening. The other common cause for feeling irritable is an emotional issue, related to feeling deprived and breaking cravings and addictions.

Remedy: Again, I refer you to the most important rule of this program—feed your hunger, and never ignore it! I cannot emphasize how critically important it is for you to keep your blood sugar levels stable. Replace old behaviors and routines with new ones. This takes conscious, deliberate, and continual effort.

Addictions and Cravings: Cravings are a gentle way of saying "addictions." Socially, we associate addictions with drugs like cocaine or heroin and behaviors like gambling, credit card spending, or pornography. So, when it comes to substances and behaviors which are more socially acceptable, like sugar, alcohol, and internet use, we dampen down our honesty and simply call the behavior cravings.

Remedy: Replace old behaviors with new, healthy ones. For example, don't turn on the television after dinner, go for a walk instead. Turn off cell phone notifications, which are major dopamine triggers. Remind yourself regularly of how well you are doing, how good you are feeling, and how good you are going to feel. Remind yourself how good it feels to be free from substances controlling you.

What Else Needs Detoxing?

Anything we do that makes us feel good, whether it is enjoying a substance like sugar or a behavior like scrolling through Facebook, stimulates a brain chemical called dopamine. Dopamine causes us to look forward to feeling good, so things that elevate this neurochemical cause us to want to repeat the behavior. In the worst case, we drive the process further by stimulating endorphins, which are the brain chemicals associated with addiction.

Dopamine and endorphin stimulation inherently is not bad at all. In fact, it is also what we do when we go for a run, lift weights, mountain bike, do yoga, meditate, or do any other behavior that makes us feel good. But it is also the chemical response in our brain when we eat sugar, drink alcohol, or use drugs like cocaine. And once given a taste of that dopamine, our neurochemistry fuels a cycle of searching to satisfy those cravings.

By choosing to go through the LivClear Detox Program you will, by default, change your dopamine secretions. Initially, this can be challenging because your subconscious is so used to getting its unhealthy way. So, there will be a struggle between your healthy self and your self-sabotaging, unhealthy self. You may have experienced this before.

You are choosing to change your lifestyle with new, healthy behaviors. These positive, self-nurturing, dopamine-stimulating changes will continue to push and pull you in a healthier direction. This is one reason the program has been designed to be 28 days, not 21 days. However, even 28 days is not long enough to create a deep-seated new habit. In 2009 the European Journal of Social Psychology published a study titled: How are habits formed: Modelling habit formation in the real world. In this research Lally and her colleagues suggested that, on average, it takes about 66 days to form a new habit. However, the time required can range from 18 to 254 days depending on the individual and the complexity of the behavior.

Detoxifying Your Choices

While the LivClear Detoxification Program focuses on the physical body, it is important to consider all the other parts of your life that will benefit from this biotransformation program. What I like about this concept is the word "bio," which derives from the Greek word *bios,* meaning one's life, course or way of living, lifetime. So, biotransformation is about transforming one's life, and it does not stop with the physical. In fact, the choices you make will have a direct effect on physical heath, and choices are always driven by beliefs, thoughts, and feelings.

Let me explain this another way. If you grew up being taught that cornflakes and milk were the perfect breakfast, this became your belief system about smart eating for the start of your day. And then, you'd go through life consuming food substances that have been altered so much and are so devoid of nutrient quality that over time they would contribute to a breakdown in your immune system, cholesterol, or microbiome, to cite a few health-related issues that might result from that typical American breakfast. And unless you question the value of these foods and explore how cornflakes and milk are processed and manufactured, consuming these substances might contribute to health problems. This is only because you believed, at one time, these foods were good for you.

There are also addictive behaviors that stimulate the production of the neurotransmitter dopamine. Dopamine causes us to feel excitement and to look forward with anticipation. We all like to continue experiencing things that bring us joy. But over time, the continued stimulation of dopamine becomes the gateway to addiction. What about news? Do you find yourself having to listen to, read, or watch a news program and feeling lost, disconnected, uninformed, and "out of it" if you don't get your dose in the morning or evening? My point is that we usually don't associate how we think or what we feel or believe with our body. But there is so much evidence showing that even the emotional state of your mother while she was carrying you in her womb can influence whether you develop obesity or mood disorders. (Clin Obstet Gynecol. 2009 September; 52(3): 425–440. doi:10.1097/GRF.0b013e3181b52df1.)

What you will be doing in this "biotransformation" program is replacing unhealthy habits with new, thoughtful, and healing behaviors which will, with practice, become your new habits. The LivClear Program starts this process by providing the foundation and navigational tools for making great changes in your body. But it is also the perfect time to expand this idea to all the other "toxic" things going on in your life. Here is a list of some of the unhealthy behaviors and habits I see in patients all the time.

- **Cell Phone Addiction**: This is HUGE and bigger than we, as a society, even realize. If possible, I'd suggest a text messaging sabbatical or at least a designated window of time where you limit the use of your phone. You can even set your messaging up to send an auto-response letting your community know you're unavailable. It is amazingly emancipating!
- **Social Media:** Facebook, Instagram, Twitter, and any of the other social media platforms you use are also designed to addict you, mislead you, stimulate negative emotions, and of course, sell you something. Do you feel good, positive, excited, and full of warm fuzzies when using these platforms? If not, then why subject yourself to such negativity?
- **Notifications:** Turn them all off! I promise, you won't miss a beat.
- **Relationships:** This is tricky because your family of origin, by its very design, has created your belief systems. Therefore, if you grew up in a dysfunctional home environment, experiencing dysfunctional parenting and relations that do not build you up,

then you simply keep repeating that which you have learned. We all do this, and sometimes it is difficult to know if a relationship is serving us well or not. And it is much more difficult to know how to fix these broken relations. We need to be surrounded by loving, positive, supportive, embracing, and nurturing people. Believe it or not, negativity can be addictive. Ask the same question: *Does this feel good or not? Does this relationship serve me well or not?*

- **News Addiction:** Next to cell phone and social media addiction, news is the most destructive, negatively charged media to which we subject ourselves. Again, ask yourself the simple question: *Do I feel better or worse after being exposed to the news?* If you do not feel empowered, validated, uplifted, or in any way positively reinforced, then why would you want to continue subjugating yourself to such mind- and heart-warping trash? Believe me, you will not miss a thing, nor will you be less informed by giving yourself a break from news for 28 days. Who knows, maybe you'll drop it forever. Personally, I have switched to reading only positive stories or those published by sources that are not funded by advertisers. *The Optimist* and *The Monitor* come to mind.

- **Watching TV or Streaming Shows/Movies:** Siting for lengthy periods in front of the television, exposing your head, heart, and subconscious to the messaging the producers, writers, and advertisers want you to experience seems like something out of Orwell's *1984*—modern-day style. Think about it, are you really being entertained by watching endless episodes of *The Most-Talked-About Series?* Again, ask yourself the same question regarding show series as you do with the news. *Do I feel better for watching it?*

- **Computer/Internet Searching:** Like cell phones, credit card charges, pornography, and a host of other dopamine-stimulating behaviors, searching the world wide web is addictive. I personally am overwhelmed whenever I am on the internet with the sheer vastness and trashiness of the information thrown at me. Though I spend most of my time on medical research sites which do not have advertising, like the NIH's PubMed, I do on occasion do general searches. It is no wonder our society is in existential crisis, as everyone, everywhere is an authority on whatever it is they are trying to sell. And how are you, a mere mortal, ever going to be able to discern untruth from useful information?

- **Video gaming:** This is an area in which I have absolutely no experience, other than watching some of my children play video games during their recreation time. These activities, just like the pings and dings of cell phones, are designed to create negative emotional reactions and dopamine spurts. It feels good and we look forward to killing bad things.

As you review most areas of our modern life, it is easy to understand that most of our unhealthy behaviors, the addictive ones, the toxic ones, are associated with screen time. It reminds me of a poignant and perspicacious forecast made by Marshall McLuhan in 1967. He was witnessing the effects of "tele-vision" on society.

"Electrical information devices for universal, tyrannical womb-to-tomb surveillance are causing a very serious dilemma between our claim to privacy and the community's need to know. The older, traditional ideas of private, isolated thoughts and actions- the patterns of mechanistic technologies- are very seriously threatened by new methods of instantaneous electric information retrieval, by the electrically computerized dossier bank- that one big gossip column that is unforgiving, unforgetful and from which there is no redemption, no erasure of early "mistakes." We have already reached a point where remedial control, born out of knowledge of media and their total effects on all of us, must be exerted. How shall the new environment be programmed now that we have become so involved with each other, now that all of us have become the unwitting workforce for social change? What's that buzzzzzzzzzzzzzzzzzzzzzzing?"

Marshall McLuhan, *The Medium is the Massage* (1967), p. 12

A Side-note About Alcohol

Alcohol is an elixir that has been used in human societies long before history was being recorded. It is found in wine, beer, and distilled liquors, and additionally, in some fermentation processes. Like most substances we consume, there is a beneficial and a harmful, or a toxic and a tolerance factor, which comes into play. This balancing act is important to understand when speaking about alcohol, because it's more damaging than many things we ingest.

Alcohol has both a water-loving component and a fat-loving component, which means it can travel easily through any water-based fluid (think blood), but also become lodged in fatty substances (think cell membranes). Alcohol can and does travel quickly through the body, potentially affecting our organs and glands.

It takes roughly sixty seconds for a blood cell to make one full cycle around the body. We experience this in the slight, gentle inebriation that we so enjoy with a glass of wine or shot of single malt. In my opinion, there is nothing really "wrong" with finding ways to relax and turn off the demands and stressors of life. We've been doing this as a species as long as we've been a species, and alcohol, for most cultures, is the go-to elixir. In the Polynesian culture, the herb kava is used in the same way, without the toxic side effects.

You could ask why eliminate it, if there is nothing "wrong" with consuming a little alcohol now and again? The real question is: Does consuming alcohol have more benefits or risks associated with its use? As with all toxins, and for that matter, all substances, we must metabolize them down to useable parts, excretable parts, or both. With alcohol, there are no real beneficial parts, except that it provides a source of fuel called acetate, which is not our preferred form. We do better burning glucose from sugars, carbohydrates, starches, and ketones, derived from fats, which is the basis of ketogenic diets.

On the contrary, alcohol produces a highly reactive metabolite called acetaldehyde, which is the chemical that causes you to feel like hungover after drinking too much. Not only does this toxin put a burden on all your organs, glands, and tissues, as evidenced in a hangover, but it is carcinogenic. Your body wants to get this toxin out as quickly as possible; however, your ability to make the enzyme acetaldehyde dehydrogenase, which clears the toxic acetaldehyde out of your body is very limited in availability. I know, it's a lot of confusing biochemistry, but just know if you drink more alcohol than you can clear out, the toxic intermediary circulates, causing all kinds of damage.

The reason you want to stop consuming alcohol during the LivClear Detoxification Program is simple—it's toxic. Here are some other reasons I'd suggest for curtailing your weekly imbibing:

- Alcohol impairs nutrient absorption in the gut by damaging the lining of your stomach and intestines.
- Alcohol interferes with nutrient absorption into the blood.
- Alcohol interferes with nutrient use in transport, storage, and excretion.
- Alcohol also causes major interruptions in your gut's microbiome.

Like many substances we enjoy in life, ask the simple question: Am I controlling _____? (Fill in the blank, in this case with alcohol). Or is it controlling me?

DAY 1

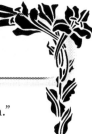

"The only impossible journey is the one you never begin."
–Tony Robbins

ISN'T THE FIRST day of a new journey exciting? And what a journey it will be! You have made an amazing decision to invest in your health, and the rewards will be limitless. The effects of the LivClear Detoxification Program will influence your mind, body, and spirit. Your rejuvenated body will function with precision, peace, and good health.

Welcome to Phase One. Enjoy your LivClear II shakes and check the Basic Dietary Guidelines. You will probably need to reference these more in the beginning, but they'll become your new health habits over time.

Always think FRESH. Fruits and vegetables, rice, nuts, and beans (maybe), nothing artificially sweetened or processed. Purchase organic whenever possible. Take extra care in choosing meats and dairy substitutes to avoid antibiotics and casein. Grass fed and free-range is best. Think mealtimes will be boring? Check the list of spices! You will be very happy.

Detox Fact: A 2014 study published in the journal, PLOS ONE, confirmed that cash register receipts contained high levels of bisphenol A. This synthetic toxic chemical has become known as a carcinogen and endocrine disruptor with a wide range of adverse health effects, including male and female infertility, as well as heart disease. Hormann AM et el: "Holding Thermal Receipt Paper and Eating Food after Using Hand Sanitizer Results in High Serum Bioactive and Urine Total Levels of Bisphenol A (BPA)," *PLOS One,* https://doi.org/10.1371/journal.pone.0110509

LivClear Detox Dosing Day 1:

Open the container of LivClear II and remove the scooper. Replace the lid and shake the LivClear II container to loosen up its contents. Take a ½ scoop twice the first day. Mix in 6 to 8 ounces of water. Pay attention to the taste and texture of the LivClear II. Drink it slowly!

Today's Tip: Add ice for a chilled treat!

Recipe: (www.ASweetLife.org)

No-Sugar-Added Baked Apples Recipe

2 apples (I used Fuji apples, but any good baking apple will do.)
½ cup of dry rolled oats
2 tablespoons of almond butter
2 teaspoons of cinnamon

Preheat oven to 425°F.

1. Wash apples and remove cores. With a paring knife, firmly place an apple on the cutting board and cut out the middle of the apple in a 360-degree motion. Watch your fingers!
2. In a small bowl, combine the oats, almond butter, and cinnamon.
3. Stuff the oats mixture into the apples and place in a baking pan.
4. Bake at 425°F for 20 minutes.
5. Let stand for 5 minutes.
6. Enjoy!

Personal Notes:

DAY 2

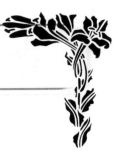

> "Nothing is impossible; the word
> itself says, "I'm POSSIBLE!"
> –Audrey Hepburn

WELCOME TO DAY 2. You're probably still feeling pretty motivated and excited since the journey is fairly new. It may seem like a long road ahead but focusing on each day as it comes is always the best way to tackle a lengthy mission.

Is your stomach feeling a bit empty? Are you confused about what to eat? Remember, you're not allowed to go hungry. You MUST feed your hunger within ten to fifteen minutes. This prevents a low blood sugar state called hypoglycemia. If this happens, you'll crave what's NOT good for you. Pay attention to your body and eat when you feel hungry. Not feeding your hunger will make this detox arduous, and it's quite the opposite. Fresh food is FUN!

Today you also get to enjoy a bit more of the LivClear II shake. We suggest that you mix it only with water for the first three days. This allows your body to fully experience LivClear II in its purity and adjust accordingly.

*If it's completely intolerable to drink LivClear II with water only, you may begin to mix it according to the mixing instructions.

Detox Fact: Pesticides are sprayed on most of the nonorganic food we consume. Unfortunately, our body easily absorbs these pesticides. That's one reason you're doing this detox. Feel like you can't afford to buy all organic food? Swapping out certain fruits that absorb the most pesticides is a good start. The "dirtiest" fruits are grapes, berries, nectarines, apples, pears, and cherries.

LivClear Detox Dosing Day 2: Take 1 full scoop and again mix it with water. Do this twice during the day.

Today's Tip: Drink your LivClear slowly! It allows for optimal absorption.

Recipe:

Bean & Spinach Soup (6 servings)

2 cups white kidney beans (cannellini), canned or home-cooked
1–2 cups kidney or red beans, canned or home-cooked
1 cup garbanzo beans (chickpeas), canned or home-cooked
2–3 cups fresh spinach or escarole, washed, drained, and chopped, or 10 ounces frozen chopped spinach
4 cups vegetable broth
2 medium onions, chopped
1 large clove garlic, minced
1 teaspoon dried basil
1 tablespoon dried parsley
1 teaspoon dried oregano
Pepper to taste

1. Wash all beans thoroughly,
2. Combine all ingredients and simmer about 45 minutes, until onions are soft.
3. Enjoy!

Personal Notes:

DAY 3

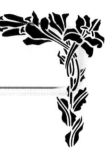

"Whether you think you can or you
think you can't, you're right."
–Henry Ford

WELCOME TO DAY 3. Your body, at this point, will begin to take a turn. Fresh foods from the dietary guidelines taste amazing, and your cravings for unhealthy, processed foods begin to diminish. Still thinking about doughnuts? Give yourself time; changes happen at slightly different rates for everyone. It WILL happen. And you CAN do it.

Is watching your spouse or children eat the unhealthy foods you think you love making your detox difficult? Try and get them involved! After all, healthy foods are beneficial for everyone. Serve a new recipe to the whole family, or simply get your kids excited about eating all the colors of the rainbow. Try and eliminate the unhealthiest foods in your household for everyone. They'll thank you later.

Day 3 is the last day we recommend enjoying your LivClear with water only. Do your best to hang in there, because tomorrow you can blend in some fruit for a delicious smoothie. Start thinking about LivClear as a meal replacement and enjoy how satisfying it is.

Detox Fact: Parabens are found in the vast majority of personal care products sold in the U.S. Check your shampoo, cleansers, and lotion. Added to prevent the growth of mold, parabens are major hormone disruptors and are linked to most female cancers.

LivClear Detox Dosing Day 3: Take 1½ scoops today, twice. You will begin sensing that this dose will satisfy your appetite, possibly substituting for a meal and definitely a snack.

Today's Tip: If necessary, you can mix LivClear II with GMO-free, unsweetened almond milk, coconut drink (not coconut water), or hemp milk for added sustenance and variety. Also, begin to read the nutrition labels on foods.

Recipe:

Tropical Salad (4–6 servings)

1 avocado, cubed
½ cup celery
8 pineapple slices, cubed
½ cup mango or pineapple juice
1 papaya or mango, cubed

1. Combine all and garnish with fresh mint leaves.
2. Enjoy!

Personal Notes:

DAY 4

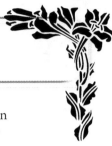

"I can't change the direction of the wind, but I can adjust my sails to always reach my destination."
–*Jimmy Dean*

WELCOME TO DAY 4. What's so great about today? Though this is not mandatory, we encourage you to start blending your LivClear II supplement into delicious smoothies. Use fruit, milk substitutes, greens—the combinations are endless. Just watch your portion sizes since all these additions do contain calories.

The LivClear II shakes will be more like meal replacements at this point, especially since you're adding nutritious ingredients. You should find that it's more than enough to fill you up. And, aren't you beginning to crave less food anyway?

After the first few days of a cleanse the fog begins to lift, energy increases, thought sharpens, sleep is deeper, and overall mood improves. If you had any doubts about committing to a cleanse, your good choices should be confirming your decision.

Detox Fact: Phthalates found in nail polish, hairspray, and synthetic fragrances are used to make products more pliable and make scents adhere to skin. They are also an endocrine disruptor and have been known to cause birth defects.

LivClear Detox Dosing Day 4: Take two full scoops twice today. Two scoops of LivClear II equals one full shake, so you will have two full shakes today. Mix according to taste and eat according to hunger from the Basic Dietary Guidelines. Remember, this is NOT a fast, so do not let yourself become hungry or, worse, ravenous!

Today's Tip: Try blending this combo with your LivClear II: 4 oz. water, 4 oz. unsweetened coconut milk, 3 ice cubes, and fresh pineapple. Side note: Pineapple can help reduce the risk of macular degeneration due to high levels of vitamin C and antioxidants.

Recipe:

Vegetarian Chili

1 tablespoon olive oil
2 tablespoons chili powder
1 medium onion, chopped
1 teaspoon cumin
2 whole carrots, diced
1 cup cooked kidney beans
4 cloves garlic, minced
1 cup cooked pinto beans
1 red bell pepper
1 28-ounce can tomatoes
1 green bell pepper
½ teaspoon freshly ground pepper
1 jalapeño pepper, fresh or canned
2 tablespoons each fresh parsley and cilantro, finely chopped

1. In large soup kettle, heat oil over low heat; add onion, carrot, garlic, and peppers.
2. Cover and cook until vegetables are soft, about 10 minutes.
3. Remove lid, add chili powder and cumin, and cook an additional 2 to 3 minutes, stirring occasionally.
4. Add beans, tomatoes, and their juice. Simmer 20 minutes.
5. Add pepper and cilantro.
6. Top bowls of chili with parsley.
7. Enjoy!

Side Note: You can also make this recipe with ground turkey, starting by browning the turkey first in the soup kettle, then continuing the recipe. This also freezes great!

Personal Notes:

DAY 5

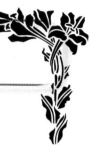

> "Believe you can and you're halfway there."
> *–Theodore Roosevelt*

WELCOME TO DAY 5. Eating this mindfully really helps us be in tune with our body. Your body tells you things every day and as the cleanse progresses, it should keep getting easier to listen.

One of the most important things to keep in mind is that we are doing a CLEANSE not a FAST. So, we want to always remind you—be sure to eat when you feel hungry! Although, you probably are finding that you don't need to eat as much or as often. Enjoy the recipes we're sharing with you and have fun creating your own.

Adjust your mindset toward food. Fresh and organic is the way to move forward, even after this cleanse is over. The more ways you discover to prepare nutritious food, the more you're likely to stick with a healthier lifestyle.

Detox Fact: Preservatives are added to nearly all processed foods, which can take a toll on how we feel every day. Studies show these additives can cause headaches, nausea, and respiratory issues. And remember, these toxicants are stored in your fatty tissues.

LivClear Detox Dosing Day 5: Take three full shakes today. Careful; this means SHAKES not SCOOPS. Remember, one shake consists of two scoops.

Today's Tip: Blend this combo with your LivClear II: 4 oz. water, 3 or 4 frozen strawberries, and ½ banana.

Recipe:

Quinoa Salad (12 servings)

1½ cup quinoa, rinsed well
¼ cup red onion, diced
3 cups vegetable broth or water

3 scallions, thinly sliced
½ cup Basic Salad Dressing
¼ cup fresh dill, chopped
1 red pepper, diced
¼ cup parsley, chopped
1 cup frozen baby peas, thawed

1. Add quinoa to broth or water in a medium saucepan, stir, and bring to a boil.
2. Reduce to simmer, then cover and cook 15 minutes without stirring or until liquid is absorbed.
3. Remove ingredients from saucepan and place in a bowl.
4. Cool slightly and toss with salad dressing and remaining ingredients.
5. Add more dressing if desired and adjust seasoning to taste.
6. Enjoy!

Basic Salad Dressing (23 servings)

¼ cup flaxseed oil (or 2 tablespoons each flaxseed and olive oils)
1–2 tablespoons lemon or lime juice
½–1 tablespoon water
1 teaspoon Dijon mustard (optional, but delicious)

1. Mix well in a shaker jar and store any leftovers in your refrigerator.
2. Pour over salad.
3. Enjoy!

*Use whole or minced garlic, oregano, basil, or other herbs of choice.

Personal Notes:

DAY 6

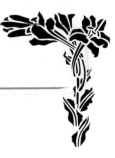

"Perfection is not attainable, but if we chase
perfection we can catch excellence."
–*Vince Lombardi*

WELCOME TO DAY 6. You're quickly approaching the height of the LivClear II consumption and feeling quite satisfied by the shakes. Isn't it surprising how filling they are?

You may also find as a result of drinking so much LivClear II that you are not as interested in food today. Again, listen to your body and pay attention to what it's telling you. If you do feel hungry, make sure you keep your blood sugar stable and eat. There's no guilt here. There's no failure if you're eating. Again, this program is a cleanse and not a fast.

At this point, you've also probably discovered a newfound love for different foods. Are you craving crunchy salads? Fresh fruit is amazing, isn't it? Who knew coconut milk and pineapple would be your new favorite combo? Take note of what you love and highlight satisfying recipes for future use.

Detox Fact: It takes about five minutes for all the blood in your body to make one full circulation, and it passes through the liver each time. One of the essential functions of the liver is to detoxify by breaking down and removing toxicants. But another important job is to filter debris from the blood. This includes the results of cellular breakdown, bacteria, yeasts, and viruses, along with their toxins.

LivClear Detox Dosing Day 6: Take four full shakes today (eight scoops total).

Today's Tip: 6 to 8 oz. water, 3 ice cubes, and one of the following: ½ apple or peach, 1 or 2 slices pineapple, or ¼ to ½ cup berries. *Did you know peaches are a great source of vitamin E, vitamin K, niacin, and copper?

Recipe:

Carrot Salad (4 servings)

2 cups carrots, shredded
½ cup celery, diced
¼ cup sunflower seeds
3–4 tablespoons light coconut milk
2 tablespoons pineapple juice

1. Mix together ingredients and chill for several hours before serving.
2. Enjoy!

Personal Notes:

PRELUDE TO NO FOOD (DAYS 7–11)

YOU HAVE SLOWLY decreased the amount of food you need each day by slowly increasing your use of the LivClear II shake. It's easier than you thought, right? This has prepared you for an incredible opportunity to really nourish and push your body toward optimum health. During days 7 through 11, you will consume as much LivClear II as you need to satisfy your hunger. By now, you understand the importance of keeping your blood sugar levels stable. This is why it is so important for you to satisfy your hunger. Only now you will do it with a shake rather than with either food or shake. The same rule applies: if you get hungry, have a shake; and you have a window of fifteen to twenty minutes to do so before your blood sugar levels drop too low.

For those of you who are in insulin resistance or have metabolic syndrome or diabetes, going without food may be challenging. It can take up to two weeks to shift your metabolism. However, I would like to emphasize again how important it is to abstain from eating. Current research shows the incredible benefits of intermittent fasting. Hypertension, weight loss, insomnia, diabetes, cancers, Alzheimer's, cognitive decline, and fatigue all improve with a reduction in the metabolic load we place on our bodies. Think reduced intake of calories while maintaining proper nutrient requirements.

Five days drinking LivClear II and not eating any foods is a win-win for you. The first benefit is that you reduce the metabolic burden on your body. When, if ever, did you go a day without taxing your digestive system with food? The second win is you will be flooding your system with the amazing nutrients needed for detoxification and energy. The third win, one we typically don't consider, is that by choosing not to eat, you break your attachments to foods and stop your addictions. This, for me, is a spiritual experience. Exercising our free will to nurture our temples enhances our relationship with God, the Divine, or however you personally define your creator.

Making the decision not to eat food, and actually going through this entire 28-day program is all about you consciously choosing to make changes. You are actually telling your subconscious mind that:

- You are worth the effort.
- You can learn new behavior.
- It isn't painful!

*Remember it is the avoidance of pain that keeps us trapped in behaviors we know are not healthy for us.

Make these five days special. Really slow down and take extra time for quiet contemplative walks or meditations. Limit your exposure to stimulation and avoid all news if that sounds appealing. Consider prayer time, and most of all, appreciate the beautiful human that you are. As a perk, if you really enjoy the no-food days, you can extend them out to a full week or even a month!

DAY 7

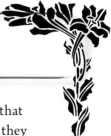

"When I was 5 years old, my mother always told me that happiness was the key to life. When I went to school, they asked me what I wanted to be when I grew up. I wrote down 'happy.' They told me I didn't't understand the assignment, and I told them they didn't understand life."
–John Lennon

WELCOME TO DAY 7. This is also the beginning of Phase Two. For the next five days, you will be at your maximum intake of LivClear II. This is also the section of the detoxification program where there is no food but LivClear II only. Giving your body rest from food is like a gift! You will regenerate and renew, allowing magic to happen internally.

Everyone is different during this stage. Some find it very easy to go without food, but some do find it difficult. Remember, feed your hunger and never ignore it. If it is hard for you, be gentle with yourself. Just because it may be challenging doesn't mean you can't have a successful experience. And just think: when you get through the next five days, won't you be proud of yourself?

This stage is all about mindset. Focus on the good you're doing for your body. Do things that make you feel happy and centered. Perhaps some gentle yoga and meditation will aid in cleansing your mind as well as your body. Never meditated before? We have some suggestions for you below.

Going five days without food is something few of us have ever done and it provides an amazing opportunity to exercise deliberate intention. It allows us to sever our ties to foods (think addictions) which frees us up spiritually, emotionally, mentally, and physically.

Detox Fact: Did you know that, according to the Natural Resources Defense Council, the drinking water of one in three Americans depends on sources that are not clearly protected from pollution? Make sure your water is clean, filtered, bottled, or otherwise uncontaminated.

LivClear Detox Dosing Day 7: Take **five full shakes** today and avoid food (two scoops per shake). Or drink as many shakes as you need during these days to satisfy your hunger.

Today's Tip: If you find that you are getting hungry soon after taking the LivClear II shake, or you simply aren't satisfied, here are some add-ons.

- Additional protein powder
- Unsweetened nut milk
- A third scoop of LivClear II

Simple Meditation For Beginners (www.Gaiam.com):

This meditation exercise is an excellent introduction to meditation techniques.

1. Sit or lie comfortably. You may even want to invest in a <u>meditation chair</u> or <u>cushion</u>.
2. Close your eyes.
3. Make no effort to control the breath; simply breathe naturally.
4. Focus your attention on the breath and on how the body moves with each inhalation and exhalation. Notice the movement of your body as you breathe. Observe your chest, shoulders, rib cage, and belly. Focus your attention on your breath without controlling its pace or intensity. If your mind wanders, return your focus back to your breath.

*Maintain this meditation practice for two to three minutes to start, and then try it for longer periods.

Personal Notes:

DAY 8

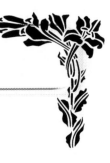

"The only person you are destined to become
is the person you decide to be."
–*Ralph Waldo Emerson*

WELCOME TO DAY 8. You should feel very proud of yourself today. It's been more than one week since you started and this is day two with no food. It's admirable that you've made such a personal commitment to yourself and stuck with it. Imagine all the other things you can accomplish when you set goals! At this point, there should be no worry that you may not be able to last through the entire 28 days. You've proved that you absolutely can.

Feeling a bit tired? This can be normal during detox. That's why getting some extra rest is so important. If possible, make sure you're getting at least eight hours of sleep at night and try to rest or nap for half an hour to an hour each day. If you find it hard to wind down before sleep, particularly during the day, there's a great breathing exercise to assist in relaxation listed below.

Detox Fact: In a 2021 published study in Frontiers in Genetics, the researchers found a relationship between gene expression and the environmental toxin bisphenol A (BSA). Their research adds to the field of study called epigenetics, which examines how environmental factors such as toxins, nutrients, and even our own thoughts and feelings govern genetic expression. In other words, only an estimated 25 percent of inherited genes dictate outcome; the majority of our genetic expression is influenced by our choices. Therefore, our environments can change our DNA. (Epigenetic Alteration Shaped by the Environmental Chemical Bisphenol A. doi: 10.3389/fgene.2020.618966)

LivClear Detox Dosing Day 8: Drink five full shakes today (two scoops per shake) and avoid food. Or drink as many shakes as you need to satisfy your hunger. Mix with water only.

Today's Tip:

Dr. Weil's 4-7-8 Breathing Exercise:

This exercise, which can be completed in five simple steps, encourages the rapid removal of carbon dioxide from your body, which aids in relaxation. Be sure to keep the tip of your tongue on the roof of your mouth right behind the front teeth.

1. Exhale completely through your mouth, making a whoosh sound.
2. Close your mouth and inhale quietly through your nose to a mental count of four.
3. Be sure to use only your diaphragm during inhalation. If uncertain, place a hand on your belly, just below your ribs. As you inhale, you should feel your belly come up under your hand.
4. Hold your breath for a count of seven. Be certain to inhale using the diaphragm only.
5. Exhale completely through your mouth, making a whoosh sound to a count of eight.
6. This is one breath. Now inhale again and repeat the cycle three more times for a total of four breaths.

Personal Notes:

DAY 9

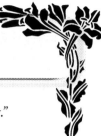

"What we achieve inwardly will change outer reality."
Plutarch

WELCOME TO DAY 9. Real changes are being made inwardly and outwardly that may surprise you. Isn't your awareness different? You may find yourself noticing more beauty in nature, valuing quiet time, and enjoying simple pleasures more than you used to. Your focus has increased and intentions are more deliberate.

Aren't you feeling lighter? Weight loss is definitely an added benefit of the LivClear cleanse, but your body's inflammation is also decreasing, which aids in lightness. Tissues that had become inflamed from those processed foods are much calmer, and your entire body is running like the clean organism it's designed to be. This would be a great time to incorporate some light yoga or gentle stretching if you haven't already done so. If yoga is new to you, it can sound intimidating, but it's actually quite the opposite. Start off with something simple like child's pose. Holding this pose for an extended period of time is both calming and rejuvenating.

Detox Fact: Did you know that formaldehyde is present in your shampoo and body wash? What's worse is that it's even put in babies' bath products. If you see ingredients like: quaternium-15, DMDM hydantoin, imidazolidinyl urea, diazolidinyl urea, sodium hydroxymethylglycinate, 2-bromo-2-nitropropane-1,3 diol (Bronopol), then it contains formaldehyde. This toxin can cause asthma, neurotoxicity, and developmental toxicity.

LivClear Detox Dosing Day 9: Drink five full shakes today (two scoops per shake) and avoid food. Mix with water only. Drink as many shakes as you need to satisfy hunger.

Today's Tip: Are you drinking enough water? Take your weight, divide it in half, and drink that many ounces per day.

Child's Pose (Popsugar.com):

- Kneel on your mat with your knees hip-width apart and your big toes touching behind you. Take a deep breath in, and as you exhale, lay your torso over your thighs. Try to lengthen your neck and spine by drawing your ribs away from your tailbone and the crown of your head away from your shoulders.
- Rest your arms beside your legs, with palms facing up, or try extending your arms out in front of you.
- Stay here for ten long breaths.

Personal Notes:

DAY 10

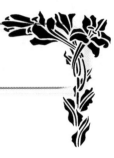

"If you don't take care of your body,
where are you going to live?"
–*Unknown*

WELCOME TO DAY 10. Doesn't that sound impressive? You've made it a whole ten days into this incredible journey and you'll be at the halfway point before you know it. If you're having trouble, and the resolve to make it through the next two days without food feels difficult, there are ways to persevere.

Have you ever tried reciting a mantra? In case you've never heard of it, a mantra is a word or saying that you repeat as a form of meditation that helps greatly with concentration. The Hindus recited Indian mantras in Sanskrit over three thousand years ago. In its simplest form, the word "Om" is repeated. This is believed to put you in tune with the rest of the universe.

Some mantras are deeply rooted in spirituality and others are simply for motivation and focus. Below, we've listed nine simple mantras (and three denominational mantras) that will help you maintain your momentum when you feel it is waning. Chose the one that speaks to you the most and try repeating it ten times.

Detox Fact (EcoWatch.com): Did you know that in farming communities there's a strong correlation between Roundup exposure and attention deficit disorder (ADHD), which is likely due to this widely used herbicides's capacity to disrupt thyroid hormone functions. By the way, Roundup is technically glyphosate.

LivClear Detox Day 10: Drink five **full shakes** today (two scoops per shake) and avoid food. Mix with water only. Drink as many shakes as you need to satisfy your hunger.

Today's Tip: Feeling a little tired? Drinking more water not only flushes out toxins, but it also increases energy and relieves fatigue.

Mantras (Sonima.com):

1. "Today, you are perfect." Jordan Younger
2. "Forward progress, just keep moving." Jamie King
3. "You are the sky. Everything else is just the weather." Pema Chodron
4. "I am attracting all the love I dream of and deserve." Candice Y. Maskell
5. "What is my path to happiness?" Tam Terry
6. "I am strong. I am beautiful. I am enough." Vanessa Pawlowski
7. "I am grateful for all that is unfolding in my life and all that is yet to come." Rachelle Tratt
8. "I am fulfilled. I am fearless." Sophia Jaffe
9. "Less is more." Robert Browning
10. "I can do all things through Christ who strengthens me." Philippians 4:13
11. "Whoever sits in the secret of the Highest will abide in the shade of *Shaddai*." Psalm 91:1.
12. "Lokah Samastah Sukhino Bhavantu." Buddhist mantra, meaning: May all beings everywhere be happy and free, and may the thoughts, words, and actions of my own life contribute in some way to that happiness and to that freedom for all.

Personal Notes:

DAY 11

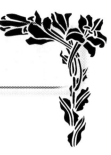

> "Garbage in, garbage out."
> *–George Fuechsel*

WELCOME TO DAY 11. This is the end of Phase Two and also your last required day without food. You're probably not even craving food as much as you anticipated. It's also nice not having to think about what you're going to eat next. More time is available for other, more meaningful things, and that aspect of your life has become simpler. In truth, abstinence is emancipating!

Perhaps this is a theme you'd like to keep in your life: simplicity. What a wonderful word. The dictionary defines it as "the quality or condition of being easy to understand or do." That sounds like a wonderful way to live. Imagine, this cleansing journey which you may have thought would be incredibly difficult has actually turned out to be an effective way to create more ease.

If you like disposing of the toxins in your body, perhaps let this spill over into other areas of your life. Maybe get rid of an obligation that causes unnecessary stress, declutter the closets in your home or make a conscious effort to let go of worry. After all, toxins can be present in many areas of our environment.

Detox Fact: Stress is quite possibly one of the most dangerous toxins. Did you know that the chemicals produced in your body by stress can turn genes on or off that regulate your immune system and the likelihood of developing cancer? In truth, stress is the greatest cause of inflammation. Chronic inflammation is the root cause of all modern diseases.

LivClear Detox Day 11: Drink five **full shakes** today (two scoops per shake) and avoid food. Mix with water only. (Reminder: if you'd like to extend the no-food days, we'll cheer you on!)

Today's Tip: Exercise is one of the best ways to lower your blood pressure, particularly a nice walk outside in nature. Breathe in the air, enjoy the sun on your face, and appreciate the beauty of whichever season is present. It's simple!

Stress Management Strategies (MayoClinic.org):

- Eating a healthy diet and getting regular exercise and plenty of sleep
- Relaxation techniques, such as yin or restorative yoga, deep diaphragm (belly) breathing, getting a massage, or learning to meditate
- Taking time for hobbies, such as reading a book, listening to music, or taking a hike in the woods
- Fostering healthy friendships
- Laughter
- Volunteering in your community
- Seeking professional counseling when needed

Personal Notes:

DAY 12

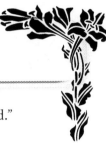

"Let food be thy medicine and medicine be thy food."
Hippocrates

WELCOME TO DAY 12. This is also the start of Phase 3. You've made it through five days without food and your body is certainly thanking you for it. However, most of us do enjoy eating real food, so now is the time we encourage you to slowly introduce certain foods back into your diet.

For the next two days, introduce fruits and vegetables only and pay attention to how you are feeling. One beautiful side effect is that your taste buds have been cleaned as has your sense of smell, so apples and bananas taste sweeter, and savory vegetables are extra satisfying. Take note of how foods taste different. Take extra time to enjoy your food; chew slowly.

Listen to your body. Things have definitely changed since you started, so take extra care to hear what your body is telling you. It may be surprising how quickly you become full, or you may crave things you never have before since your body is ridding itself of toxins—particularly sugar. If you accidentally eat a bit too much, take note and do a little less next time.

Detox Fact: Did you know that berries are part of the Dirty Dozen? "The Dirty Dozen" is a term used to list fruits and veggies that are more likely to have higher environmental pesticides and herbicides which are commercially, not organically grown. It is a term and list compiled by organizations like the Environmental Working Group (EWG) It's often difficult to afford all-organic produce when you go grocery shopping, but certain fruits and vegetables contain higher levels of pesticides because of the chemicals applied to them before and after harvest. Berries contain some of the highest levels, so if it's within your budget to go organic, then blueberries, strawberries, and raspberries are a great place to start.

LivClear Detox Day 12: Take **four full shakes** (two scoops each) these two days and begin adding food back into your routine from the Basic Dietary Guidelines.

Today's Tip: Blueberries are a great source of vitamin C, potassium, sodium, and fiber. They contain several acids, including oxalic, malic acid, and citric acid. They also contain anthocyanidins, which may explain the effectiveness of blueberries in the treatment of urinary tract infections.

Recipe:

Blueberry Green Smoothie

½ apple
4 ice cubes
½ cup fresh blueberries
¼ cup water
1 cup raw spinach

Blend together and enjoy!

Personal Notes:

DAY 13

"Don't eat anything your great-great grandmother wouldn't recognize as food. There are a great many food-like items in the supermarket your ancestors wouldn't recognize as food . . . stay away from these."
–Michael Pollan

WELCOME TO DAY 13. How wonderful do those fruits and veggies taste? It's almost as if you don't even need anything else. This is a great time to make a conscious shift in your life to make produce the bulk of your diet. Try and eat foods the color of the rainbow every day. These fresh foods are nutrient rich, delicious, and so satisfying.

Enjoy your last day of fruits and veggies only, and make yourself a nice, crunchy salad. Also, review your guidelines in preparation for tomorrow when you can start adding in some additional food. A delicious dressing, perhaps?

Wondering what's actually happening in your body at this point? Neutralized toxins, now made water-soluble, are removed from the body in the urine via the kidneys or in the bile/feces through the intestinal tract. Pretty interesting stuff!

Detox Fact: Leafy greens like lettuce and kale are among the most likely vegetables to retain pesticide contamination. To remove most of the pesticides, remove the outer leaves, then wash. Soak the washed leaves in a sea salt solution for five to ten minutes, and then repeat.

LivClear Detox Day 13: Take **four full shakes** (two scoops each) these two days and begin adding food back into your routine from the Basic Dietary Guidelines.

Today's Tip: Think you know about kale? It's a garden vegetable originally cultivated in the Mediterranean region. An important crop in Roman times, it became a staple food among peasants during the Middle Ages. This leafy green was brought to the United States from England in the 17th century.

Kale is one of the heartiest members of the cabbage family. An excellent source of vitamins A and C and of potassium, it is also a good source of vitamin B6, copper, folic acid, calcium, iron, thiamine, riboflavin, niacin, and zinc. Whew!

Recipe:

Kale and Pink Grapefruit Salad (www.Bonappetit.com)

1 pink grapefruit
2 tablespoons olive oil (or omit the oil and only use a squeeze of grapefruit/lemon juice)
Kosher salt and freshly ground black pepper
8 cups thinly sliced kale (center ribs and stems removed)
1 avocado, halved, pitted, and sliced into half-inch wedges

1. Using a sharp knife, cut peel and white pith from grapefruit; discard.
2. Working over a small bowl, cut between membranes to release segments into bowl. Squeeze juice from membranes into another small bowl; add any accumulated juices from bowl with segments (there should be about ¼ cup juice total).
3. Whisk oil into juice.
4. Season to taste with salt and pepper.
5. Place kale in a large bowl and drizzle 3 tablespoons of dressing over.
6. Toss to combine and let stand for 10 minutes while kale wilts slightly.
7. Toss once more, then arrange grapefruit segments and avocado slices over kale.
8. Drizzle with remaining dressing and serve.
9. Enjoy!

Personal Notes:

DAY 14

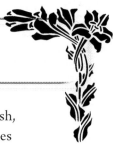

"Everybody today seems to be in such a terrible rush,
anxious for greater developments and greater riches
and so on, so that children have very little time for their
parents. Parents have very little time for each other, and in
the home begins the disruption of the peace of the world."
–Mother Teresa of Calcutta

WELCOME TO DAY 14. Today, your food options widen a bit. For the next two days you may begin adding nuts, seeds, beans, and legumes into your diet, along with fruits and vegetables. You'll be amazed with what you can do with just these additions!

By reintroducing these foods, you're adding a significant amount of protein and fiber back into your diet. A little bit goes a long way, and you probably need less than you think to feel full. In fact, surveys suggest that Americans consume nearly 1½ to almost double the amount of recommended protein per day, but unfortunately, it is the wrong kind of protein. Animal protein, especially from beef, pork, and lamb, should be a staple of your diet. But it must be from animals that are humanely raised and allowed to graze and live in a free range. The protein, and especially the fat in this protein, is what your body needs and is accustomed to from the thousands of years we've walked this planet. Commercial-grade meats and poultry are high in omega-6 fatty acids, which, in excess, don't make good cell membranes or structures. So, clean-sourced proteins and organic veggies should be your mantra!

Detox Fact: We tend to think of peanuts and peanut butter as a healthy staple in our diet, but peanuts are actually a very moldy nut. They are loaded with aflatoxins, which is a fancy word for fungus poop. Who wants a PB&J now? Yuck!

LivClear Detox Day 14: Take **three full shakes** today (two scoops each).

Today's Tip: Pumpkin seeds are quite the tiny powerhouse. They are packed with magnesium, protein, copper, and zinc. They are also rich in antioxidants, which are beneficial all around. They're extra good for your heart and immune system. So, whenever you feel you need a boost, reach for pumpkin seeds.

Recipe:

Strawberry Pumpkin Seed Smoothie (www.TheFullHelping.com)

1 cup frozen strawberries
¾ cup almond milk
2 tablespoons pumpkin seeds
2 scoops of LivClear (to be substituted with 1 scoop of protein powder when you're not cleansing)
1 handful of raw spinach
1 teaspoon cinnamon

Blend and enjoy!

Personal Notes:

DAY 15

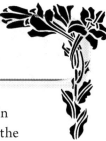

"As human beings, our greatness lies not so much in
being able to remake the world—that is the myth of the
atomic age—as in being able to remake ourselves."
–Mahatma Gandhi

WELCOME TO DAY 15. How are you feeling today? Pretty great, we bet.
While your body is still continuing to get rid of toxins, you're more in a stage
of reprogramming. Now that most of the junk is gone, this reintroduction
process is teaching your body a new way of eating. One that you'll enjoy for
a lifetime.

Want to hear another bit of great news? You're officially past the halfway
point in the LivClear cleanse. In fact, the difficult part is far behind you, and
it only gets easier from here.

Hopefully, you're also enjoying eating beans, nuts, seeds, and legumes.
There are a TON of great recipes available that offer creative ways to use
these nutrition-packed nuggets in virtually every meal of the day. We list one
of our favorite salads below.

Detox Fact: Are you reaching for canned beans? It's been found that the
BPA (bisphenol A) in epoxy resins found in the lining of metal cans can leach
into your food. BPA has been linked to hypertension, aggression, obesity,
and cancer. Although it's not as convenient, dried beans are significantly
safer. Always be on the lookout for BPA on food labels.

LivClear Detox Day 15: Take **three full shakes** today (two scoops each).
A side note here: many patients going through the program ask if they can
continue with three shakes per day and one meal for an extended period. We
will be your greatest cheerleader if you do!

Today's Tip: Getting bored with plain water? Get a big pitcher of water and
add things like orange slices, lemon, lime, watermelon, cucumber, and even
mint. Your favorite fresh flavors will make it easier to keep up the sipping.

Recipe:

Black Bean Salad (4 servings)

2 cups black beans, cooked
1 cup cherry tomatoes
¼ cup red onion, chopped
½ cup red or yellow bell pepper, chopped
1 tablespoon olive oil
1 teaspoon lemon or lime juice
1–2 teaspoons cumin

1. Combine ingredients in a bowl.
2. Chill before serving.
3. Enjoy!

Personal Notes:

DAY 16

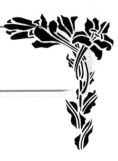

"You are not a drop in the ocean. You
are the entire ocean in a drop."
—*Rumi*

WELCOME TO DAY 16. The adventure of adding another food group back into your diet continues. If starches like rice, oats, millet, quinoa, amaranth, teff, tapioca, and buckwheat are allowed in your program, begin to enjoy them in moderation. This can include pasta, bread, crackers, flours, etc. Be sure to keep them gluten-free, organic, and whole whenever possible. Whole grain, organic basmati white rice is the best. Check to be sure any gluten-free product you use are non-GMO, as these foods are most always prepared with GMO products. Look for the non-GMO label!

Grains are not tolerated well by most of us, as their macronutrient mix is different from any other food we enjoy. This category of foods typically causes the greatest reaction when added back into your diet, so start off with small amounts and pay attention to how your body reacts. Often, concentrated carbohydrates are emotional "trigger" foods as well. Being aware of these factors and beginning slowly with limited portions should be enough for successful reintroduction. And if you know you do tolerate some nongluten grains, then it is best to have them in the later part of the day.

Detox Fact: Parboiled rice (like Minute Rice) can contain aflatoxins, which are produced by certain mold and fungus. High levels of humidity foster the growth of these mold and fungus, causing elevated levels of these toxins that lead to contamination.

LivClear Detox Day 16: Take **two full shakes** today (two scoops each).

Today's Tip: Jasmine or basmati rice (which are both varieties of brown rice) still have their germ and bran layers. This means they retain nutrient-rich benefits like B vitamins, phosphorus, and magnesium. Organic is always best.

Recipe:

Nutty Green Rice (4 servings)

1 cup brown basmati rice
2 cups water
1½ tablespoons lemon juice
1½ tablespoons olive oil
½ cup almonds
½ cucumber, diced
½ small bunch of parsley
1 clove of garlic
Salt and pepper to taste

1. Bring water to a boil and add rice.
2. Stir, then simmer, covered, for 45 minutes (do not stir again).
3. Remove from heat and let sit for another 10 minutes, then remove cover and allow to cool.
4. While rice is cooking, blend almonds, parsley, garlic, oil (or water), and lemon juice in a food processor.
5. When rice is cool, stir in the nut mixture and add cucumber.
6. Salt and pepper to taste.
7. Enjoy!

Personal Notes:

DAY 17

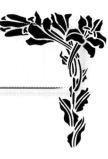

> "In order to change we must be sick and
> tired of being sick and tired."
> *–Fannie Lou Hamer 1964*

WELCOME TO DAY 17. We hope you're still enjoying starches in your diet, but be sure to watch out for any gluten-containing product. Wheat, corn, rye, barley, spelt, kamut, and oats all fall into this category. So, while you may be excited for pasta, just be sure it's gluten-free.

If weight loss is your goal, we recommend going minimal on the starches or eliminating them completely. If you're going to include some starch, it's best to go with natural starches like root vegetables, brown rice, beans, and peas. Refined starches like crackers, cereal, baked goods, and bread should be avoided or eaten sparingly.

Refined starches have had most of their nutrients and fiber stripped out. Since they're digested so quickly, they cause spikes in blood sugar and insulin levels. They can often leave you feeling hungry soon after eating, which may lead to overeating. So, choose your carbs wisely, eat in moderation, and be sure to include some protein.

Detox Fact (thehealthyhomeeconomist.com): Common wheat harvesting protocol in the United States is to drench the wheat fields with the herbicide Roundup several days before the combine harvesters work through the fields. This practice, known as desiccation, allows for an earlier, easier, and bigger harvest. Pre-harvest application of Roundup or other herbicides containing the deadly active ingredient glyphosate to wheat and barley as a desiccant was suggested as early as 1980. Since 2002, it has become routine in the conventional farming community to use these products as a drying agent seven to ten days before harvest. Other research suggests the real culprit in wheat, causing gluten intolerance for so many, is NOT the gluten but the glyphosate.

LivClear Detox Day 17: Take **two full shakes** today (two scoops each).

Today's Tip: Even in the medical literature there is confusion about whether oats should be avoided because of gluten. Oats have a storage protein, avenin, which is part of the gluten family of proteins, so it is similar to those found in wheat but does not cause the same kind of damage and inflammation as glutens from wheat. The consensus is—maybe! So, if you're really sensitive to wheats, rye, and barley, then stay away from oats. The other issue with oats is cross contamination with gluten from wheat from their manufacturing facility.

Recipe:

Pasta and Beans (4 servings)

16 ounce can white beans
3 tablespoons olive oil, divided (use water substitute for cooking vegetables if you're eliminating oil)
2 onions, chopped
2 carrots chopped
1 teaspoon dried oregano
2 tablespoon dried basil
16-ounce can tomatoes or 4 tomatoes peeled and chopped
½ cup bean liquid
1–2 teaspoons salt
½ lb. rice, red lentil, or chickpea elbow pasta

1. Drain beans, reserving liquid.
2. Heat 1–2 tablespoons olive oil in heavy casserole dish.
3. Add onions, carrots, oregano, and basil; cook until vegetables are wilted.
4. Add tomatoes, bean liquid, and salt and pepper to taste.
5. Cover and simmer for about 10 minutes until the vegetables are tender.
6. Add the drained beans and simmer for another 10 minutes.
7. Meanwhile, cook and drain the macaroni.
8. Toss with 1 tablespoon more olive oil, and then mix with the bean sauce.
9. Enjoy!

Personal Notes:

DAY 18

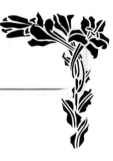

"It is better to conquer yourself than
to win a thousand battles."
–Buddha

WELCOME TO DAY 18. Only ten days left, and what a beautiful journey it has been. However, even when the full 28 days is complete, you will most certainly want to continue the good new habits you've been practicing mentally and physically.

At this time, you can reintroduce the final food group, which is protein. Foods that fall into this category contain all the essential amino acids and include all meats, poultry, fish, eggs, and dairy. But since you're still cleansing, there are some restrictions. Continue to omit dairy, commercial beef and pork, eggs, and shellfish. These foods have a higher likelihood of causing an allergic reaction and/or inflammation in the body.

Concentrated proteins that are allowed are fresh and water-packed fish, chicken, turkey, wild game, and free-range beef, pork and lamb. If you have access to organically-raised, grass-fed, free-range, uncontaminated sources of beef and pork, please enjoy them.

Detox Fact: Chickens that are farmed in large factories are stressed out. This makes them more susceptible to illness, which is rampant in overcrowded facilities. As a result, they are given more antibiotics that eventually wind up in the bodies of the humans who consume them. Over time, this contributes to our antibiotic resistance.

LivClear Detox Day 18: Take **two full shakes** today (two scoops each).

Today's Tip: Try to add greens like spinach to your smoothies whenever possible. Worried it may not taste good? The sweetness of fruit overpowers the flavor of greens. As long as you have a sweet fruit like pineapple or strawberries, you'll never know the greens are there.

Recipe:

Curried Chicken Salad (4 servings)

2½ lbs. boneless, skinless white meat chicken
½ cup mango or papaya juice
1 cup red or green apple, unpeeled and diced
1 teaspoon curry powder
2 stalks celery, diced
¼ teaspoon turmeric
1 tablespoon olive oil
½ small jicama, peeled and diced (optional)
Salt and pepper to taste

1. Bake chicken at 350°F for 20 minutes, then dice.
2. Place cooked, diced chicken in a large salad bowl and cool.
3. Combine with remaining ingredients.
4. Adjust seasoning to taste and refrigerate for an hour before serving.
5. Enjoy!

Personal Notes:

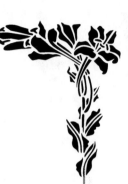

DAY 19

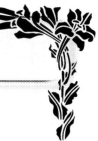

> "To eat is a necessity, but to eat intelligently is an art."
> –La Rochefoucald

WELCOME TO DAY 19. Wondering what to eat? A great answer is SOUP! Think about what most soups are made of. They're packed with vegetables and are "souper" hydrating (see what we did there?).

The best part is they're easy to make. Try and stay away from canned soups when possible because of toxins from the metal cans and the high sodium content. Once you realize how easy it is to make homemade soup, you'll be doing it all the time. We love making extra to freeze for another meal. Consider investing in an Instant Pot, which is an amazing cooking tool based on pressure-cooking technology.

Think about your favorite vegetables and center your soups around those. Carrots, peppers, onions, celery—the list is endless. You'd be hard pressed to find a vegetable that doesn't taste great in soup. Stay away from using cream and stick to a good stock. Remember the rainbow!

Detox Fact: Are you missing an evening glass of wine, your thirst-quenching beer, or a de-stressing cocktail? Alcohol is one of the most toxic substances we can put into our precious bodies. It causes numerous diseases, including cancer, and, according to a recent study in *The Lancet*, it offers no nutritional value.

LivClear Detox Day 19: Take **two full shakes** today (two scoops each).

Today's Tip: Did you know that green beans are not only a great source of fiber but also high in protein? They are also packed with vitamins A, C, K, and B6, folic acid, calcium, silicon, iron, manganese, potassium, and copper. Talk about nutrient rich!

Recipe:

Minestrone Soup (8 servings)

1 tablespoon olive oil
⅓ cup brown rice
1 large onion, chopped
3 carrots, sliced or diced
2 cloves garlic, minced
1 bay leaf
6 cups vegetable stock or water
2 stalks celery, chopped
1 28-ounce can diced or crushed tomatoes
1 16-ounce can kidney beans or 2 cups home-cooked
1 lb. fresh green beans cut into 1-inch pieces or
10-ounce package frozen cut green beans

1. In soup kettle or pot, sauté onion, celery, carrots, and garlic until softened.
2. Add stock or water, tomatoes, rice, and bay leaf.
3. Bring to a boil and cover, reducing heat to a simmer for 50 minutes; stir occasionally.
4. Stir in kidney beans and green beans, and simmer for 5–10 minutes more until all vegetables are tender.
5. Remove bay leaf before serving.
6. Enjoy!

Personal Notes:

DAY 20

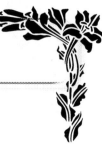

> "Yesterday I was clever, so I wanted to change the
> world. Today I am wise, so I am changing myself."
> *–Rumi*

WELCOME TO DAY 20. At this point, you're so used to eating clean-sourced proteins and fresh fruits and vegetables that you probably can't imagine a day without them. Think about your previous lifestyle and what brought you to this cleanse. Those less desirable habits are merely a distant memory.

Now that you're obsessed with fruits and vegetables, have you ever thought of planting a garden? Perhaps you already have one, but if you don't, there are a ton of options that are much easier than you think. You'd be hard pressed to find a better feeling than eating a salad made from vegetables that you grew yourself and were FREE.

You can dedicate a small, sunny patch in your yard, construct a raised garden, or simply use a pot if you have limited space. Vegetables like radishes, spinach, and peppers are extremely easy to grow. With just a few Google searches, you can find a plethora of information to get you started. Get growing!

Detox Fact: Washing your fruits and vegetables can greatly reduce the amount of pesticide residue from your food, but it's impossible to get rid of it completely. Pesticides are absorbed through the roots and end up in the tissue of the fruit or vegetable. Avoid pesticides all together by buying certified organic whenever possible or grow your own.

LivClear Detox Day 20: Take **two full shakes** today (two scoops each).

Today's Tip: Chickpeas are great at controlling blood sugar levels and appetite. They're full of fiber and nutrients. Hummus is a great way to eat chickpeas but be careful. Watch your portions and avoid excess calories and fat. When making your own hummus, don't skimp on the parsley. It's great for your gut, which is where your immune system is located

Recipe:

Hummus (6 servings)

2 cups canned garbanzo beans (chickpeas), washed, or home-cooked
⅓ cup lemon juice
2 tablespoons olive oil
1 teaspoon cumin
2 cloves garlic, crushed
¼ cup tahini
Paprika, sea salt, and fresh parsley to taste

1. Drain beans and reserve liquid.
2. Blend beans with remaining ingredients.
3. If mixture seems dry, add some of the reserved liquid slowly to the blender to make a smooth paste.
4. Garnish with a sprinkle of paprika and parsley.
5. Enjoy!

Personal Notes:

DAY 21

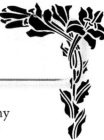

> "The best six doctors anywhere and no one can deny
> it are sunshine, water, rest, air, exercise, and diet."
> *–Wayne Fields*

WELCOME TO DAY 21. Feeling fabulous? We thought so. Even though you're already feeling pretty great, let's step it up a notch. One of our favorite activities is spending time outdoors. Sunshine can do amazing things for your health.

The Mayo Clinic supports that getting anywhere from five to fifteen minutes of sunlight on your arms, hands, and face two to three times a week is enough to enjoy the vitamin D-boosting benefits of the sun. Not only is vitamin D a major serotonin booster, but it plays an important role in bone health. Low vitamin D levels have been linked to rickets in children and osteoporosis in adults.

While we all know that overexposure can lead to skin cancer, a study from Environmental Health Perspectives found that moderate sun exposure reduces your chances of getting colon cancer, Hodgkin's lymphoma, ovarian cancer, pancreatic cancer, or prostate cancer. Research shows that sunlight is also a potential treatment for rheumatoid arthritis, lupus, inflammatory bowel disease, and thyroiditis. So, whether it's gardening, a nice walk, or a brisk run, getting outside has unlimited benefits!

Detox Fact: While no method is 100 percent effective in removing pesticides, washing your apples in a mixture of one teaspoon of baking soda and two cups of water is the most effective at removing residue. A CNN study found that pesticides break down faster in baking soda.

LivClear Detox Day 21: Take **two full shakes** today (two scoops each).

Today's Tip: Apples are a great source of potassium and vitamin C. They contain pectin, which helps to control cholesterol, blood sugar, and cellulose levels, as well as improving intestinal function. Because most of the apple's nutrients are concentrated just under the skin, it is best to eat it unpeeled and organic. While they are not a miracle cure, apples do have a number of medicinal properties, hence the popular saying, "An apple a day keeps the doctor away."

Recipe:

Red Cabbage-Apple Salad (6 servings)

1 small head red cabbage, coarsely chopped
2 green onions, chopped
1 stalk celery, chopped
10 radishes, sliced
¼ cup walnuts, chopped
1–2 tablespoons lemon juice
3 tart green apples, unpeeled, washed & diced
Dash of garlic

Mix everything in a serving bowl and let sit for an hour, stirring once or twice. Enjoy!

Personal Notes:

DAY 22

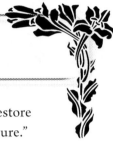

"No matter how much it gets abused, the body can restore balance. The first rule is to stop interfering with nature."
–*Deepak Chopra*

WELCOME TO DAY 22 You're doing a fantastic job allowing your body to cleanse itself. In fact, our bodies are cleansing all the time. One of the main organs that aids in detoxifying is the liver. Since it's such a vital organ, we want to make sure we keep it healthy.

There are some easy dos and don'ts that will keep your liver in tip-top shape. DON'T consume much alcohol, take medications like Tylenol (acetaminophen) in moderation, and be careful about breathing in harmful toxins from insecticides or cleaning products. DO eat a healthy diet, get regular exercise, and drink coffee. Yes! You read that correctly. Some early research suggests that drinking coffee can lower your risk of getting liver disease. The only caveat is to avoid espresso and French pressed coffees as they contain the diterpenes cafestol and kahweol. Both affect cholesterol but can be filtered out with paper. ALWAYS use organic, as coffee is ranked as one of the most chemically treated crops.

Detox Fact: According to the Environmental Working Group, "One toxic insecticide widely used in banana production is chlorpyrifos, a potent neuro-toxicant member of the organophosphate insecticide family. Chlorpyrifos can harm workers, communities, and the environment but is not generally detected on peeled bananas. Children are especially sensitive to chlorpyrifos toxicity. The chemical can disrupt brain development and impair cognitive functions, measured by intelligence tests, when the child is exposed during pregnancy and early childhood. Costa Rican researchers found that children living near banana fields where pesticides were used had much higher concentrations of chlorpyrifos in their bodies than children living where only 12 percent of farmers reported using pesticides." (Reference: https://www.ewg.org/news-insights/news/how-avoid-brain-damaging-chlorpyrifos)

LivClear Detox Day 22: Take **two full shakes** today (two scoops each).

Today's Tip: As a banana ripens, the sugars in it are transformed. Initially present as starch, which is difficult to digest, they gradually convert into sugars, such as fructose, glucose, and sucrose, which are easily assimilated. This explains why a green banana is difficult to digest, while an overripe banana is so sweet and nourishing. A great source of vitamin B6, potassium, vitamin C, riboflavin, folic acid, and magnesium, they can also be a mild laxative when overripe.

Recipe:

Bulletproof Coffee (Original by Dave Asprey)

1 cup brewed organic coffee
1 teaspoon to 2 tablespoons MCT oil
1–2 tablespoons grass-fed, unsalted butter or 1--2 teaspoons grass-fed ghee

1. Brew 1 cup (8–12 ounces) of organic coffee.
2. Add coffee, MCT oil, and butter or ghee to a blender, or use a handheld emulsifier directly in your coffee cup.
3. Blend 20–30 seconds until it looks creamy
4. Enjoy!

Personal Notes:

DAY 23

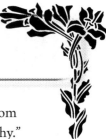

"Your body holds deep wisdom. Trust in it. Learn from it. Nourish it. Watch your life transform and be healthy."
−Erin Keane

WELCOME TO DAY 23. Up to this point, you've read a lot about food. You know what you should eat and how much you should be eating. We've also been reminding you to listen to your body. If these things seem difficult, there's a really easy way to merge the two thoughts, it's called EATING MINDFULLY.

When you eat mindfully or intuitively, you're letting your body lead the way. You're creating a healthy relationship with food and learning what your body really needs. Does this sound vague? It's actually pretty simple.

First off, when you're eating, turn off all distractions and actually pay attention to what's going in your mouth. Be mindful of when you're actually hungry and pay attention to when you stop feeling hungry. Think about how certain foods will make you feel. Will this make me feel good and energized after I eat it or will I feel sluggish and tired? Lastly, be aware of why you're eating. Are you bored, tired, or sad? If it's emotional hunger you're feeling, find something else fulfilling instead of food. Save the food for actual hunger!

Detox Fact: "According to the USDA's Pesticide Data Program, 35 different pesticides have been found on conventional potatoes. The chemical that is found on 76 percent of all conventional potatoes is chlorpropham, a herbicide that is used to stop the growth of weeds and inhibit potato sprouting." (LivingMaxwell.com)

LivClear Detox Day 23: Take **two full shakes** today (two scoops each).

Today's Tip: Root vegetables easily absorb pesticides, but when you buy organic sweet potatoes, you can rest assured they were grown sustainably and did not receive any chemical baths. Sweet potatoes contain more potassium than bananas and nearly half of your daily recommended value of vitamin C.

Recipe:

Instant Pot Chicken No-Tortilla Soup (Unbound Wellness)

2 tablespoons avocado oil
1 onion, diced
1 jalapeño, diced and seeded
3 cloves garlic, minced
2 medium zucchinis, chopped (about 2 cups)
4 cups chicken broth
1 15-ounce can fire-roasted tomatoes
Juice of one lime
1 teaspoon sea salt
½ teaspoon black pepper
1 teaspoon cumin
2 teaspoon oregano
1 lb. chicken breast
2 tablespoons cilantro
1–2 medium avocados, sliced

1. Set the Instant Pot to sauté and add the avocado oil.
2. Once heated, add the onion, jalapeño, and garlic.
3. Cook for 3–4 minutes or until the onion is slightly translucent.
4. Add the zucchini, and sauté for another 1–2 minutes to soften.
5. Pour in the broth, tomato, lime juice, chicken, and seasonings (reserving cilantro to serve), and stir well to combine.
6. Hit cancel on the Instant Pot and place the lid on with the valve sealed. Set the Instant Pot to high pressure for 12 minutes.
7. Allow to come to pressure and cook. Quick-release the pressure and carefully remove the lid. Use a meat thermometer to ensure the chicken is 165°F. Set the Instant Pot to sauté for longer if needed.
8. Pull the chicken out and shred with two forks. Add back to the soup and stir.
9. Serve topped with cilantro, avocado, and additional lime juice to taste.
10. Enjoy!

Personal Notes:

DAY 24

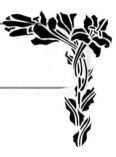

> "There is no one giant step that does
> it. It's a lot of little steps."
> *—Unknown*

WELCOME TO DAY 24. I'm sure you've learned so many little steps along this journey to improve your overall health. One of the best things you can do for yourself is a daily walk—even if the weather is less than desirable. This can help you maintain a healthy weight and prevent heart disease, high blood pressure, and type 2 diabetes.

But how much is enough? Studies show that if you don't get at least 5,000 steps per day, over time, your health will suffer. You need at least 7,500 per day for it to be considered exercise. Reaching 10,000 per day can help you lose up to one pound per week. A group of postal workers in the UK were given trackers to wear for an entire week, and those who walked over 15,000 steps per day showed almost no risk for cardiovascular disease.

While walking 15,000 steps per day sounds wonderful, it would take the average person around 3½ hours, which is impractical for most working adults. But it is a great idea to try out a fitness tracker and see how much you're actually moving. The results will probably surprise you and hopefully motivate you to increase the number of steps you take each day. Remember, some is always better than none.

(Reference:Banach MJ. et el. The association between daily step count and all-cause and cardiovascular mortality: a meta-analysisEuropean Journal of Preventive Cardiology (2023) 00, 1–11://doi.org/10.1093/eurjpc/zwad229)

Detox Fact: Watch out for talc in your personal care products (particularly powdery makeup like eye shadow and blush). During the mining process, it can be contaminated with asbestos fibers, causing respiratory issues and several cancers.

LivClear Detox Day 24: Take **two full shakes** today (two scoops each).

Today's Tip: When choosing personal care products, look for companies you can trust to manufacture their products sustainably without any toxins. Some of our favorites are Beauty Counter, Pacifica, and Ilia. You'll find you like their performance just as much as what you were using before and eliminating these toxins will reduce inflammation in your body.

Recipe:

Baked Apple with Nut Topping (4 servings)

4 firm cooking apples (Granny Smith, McIntosh, etc.)
½ cup raw walnut or almond pieces
8 tablespoons raisins
Cinnamon to taste
Pure vanilla extract

1. With a knife, cut apples horizontally around the middle to keep the skin from splitting during baking.
2. Core apples and fill the center of each with 2 tablespoons raisins.
3. Sprinkle with cinnamon.
4. Bake at 350°F for 45 minutes, or until tender.
5. While apples are baking, whirl walnuts or almonds (must be raw to get creamy) in a blender, adding water gradually until you get the consistency you prefer. (The longer you blend, the smoother the mixture becomes.)
6. Add a few drops of pure vanilla extract for extra flavor.
7. Spoon over hot apples.
8. Enjoy!

Personal Notes:

DAY 25

"Those who think they have no time for healthy eating …
will sooner or later have to find time for illness."
−*Edward Stanley*

WELCOME TO DAY 25. After detoxifying your system for the past twenty-five days, I'm sure you can fully believe that food is medicine. Health in = beneficial outcome; less healthy = less desirable outcome.

Nutrient deficiencies and toxicity from a poor diet are linked to nearly all modern health conditions. A study done by researchers at the Comprehensive Cancer Center, Baylor College of Medicine, 50% percent of cancer patients are believed to be malnourished. While a healthy diet is no guarantee that you'll never be affected by disease, it does significantly decrease the odds. (Reference: Journal of Geriatric Oncology 10 (2019) 763–769)

It's no surprise that organic raw vegetables top the list of food that acts as medicine for your body. They restore the body's pH and detoxify the blood while being very low in calories. A little-known fact is that the antioxidants in vegetables help protect the plant from harsh environmental factors, and when we consume them, we reap the same benefits.

Detox Fact: According to Natural Health News, higher levels of fluoride in drinking water appear to be associated with an increased risk for hypothyroidism. Locations with fluoridated water were more than 30 percent more likely to have high levels of hypothyroidism, compared to areas with low fluoride levels in their water. In fact, all of Western Europe has banned water fluoridation because they believe it's immoral to medicate their population without their consent.

LivClear Detox Day 25: Take **2 full shakes** today (2 scoops each).

Today's Tip: If you'd like to drink water in its purest form, the top 3 filters are reverse osmosis, deionizers, and activated alumina. These filters remove up to 90 percent of fluoride and other toxins. Activated carbon filters do not.

Just be aware that when you remove this much unhealthy stuff, you're also removing good stuff, too, like essential minerals from your water.

Recipe:

Sweet Potato Squash Delight (4–6 servings)

1 medium butternut squash, cut into chunk
½ teaspoon ginger
2 medium sweet potatoes, cut into chunks
½ teaspoon cinnamon
Dash of nutmeg
¼ cup of almond milk

1. Preheat oven to 350°F.
2. Steam squash and sweet potato until tender.
3. Remove peels, and purée in food processor.
4. Add ginger, cinnamon, nutmeg, and almond milk (add enough to match the consistency of mashed potatoes).
5. Put mixture into 1½ qt. casserole dish, and garnish with a sprinkle of cinnamon.
6. Bake about 15 minutes.
7. Enjoy!

Personal Notes:

DAY 26

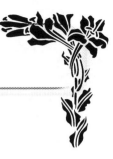

"The natural healing force in each one of us
is the greatest force in getting well."
—*Hippocrates*

WELCOME TO DAY 26. Do you know how happy your gut is? By eliminating gluten and a host of antigenic foods from your diet, you've given your digestive tract a huge break and opportunity to repair itself. Your good bacteria are flourishing and immunity is on the rise!

Vegetables, particularly greens like broccoli, cabbage, and kale, have sulfur-containing metabolites called glucosinolates, which reduce inflammation and remove harmful pathogens from the gastrointestinal tract. This keeps your bowels happy, too. Symptoms of an unhealthy gut can include indigestion, gas and bloat, constipation or diarrhea, GERD, and any combination of these.

When the gut is put back into balance you can eliminate health issues like acne and skin rashes, allergies, brain fog, insomnia, chronic fatigue, headaches, yeast infections, and, of course, weight gain. Most people don't realize the importance of a healthy gut. It's like the gatekeeper of your entire body, including the brain. Keep it happy, and almost everything else will be in good working order.

Detox Fact: According to Consumer Reports, studies have linked long-term pesticide exposure to increased risk of Alzheimer's and Parkinson's disease, and prostate, ovarian, and other cancers, as well as depression and respiratory problems. Green beans, sweet bell peppers, and hot peppers are veggies that Consumer Reports says shoppers should always buy organic. Buying vegetables grown in Mexico, South America and Guatemala can be especially risky. All the more reason to purchase your vegetables locally and organically.

LivClear Detox Day 26: Take **two full shakes** today (two scoops each).

Today's Tip: Dry methods of cooking like roasting, grilling, and stir-frying help your vegetables retain more nutrients. And they're much tastier, too!

Recipe:

Oven-Roasted Veggies

1. Use any combination of the following, cut into bite-sized pieces; unpeeled and washed eggplant, small sweet potatoes, yellow or green summer squash, asparagus, and peeled red onion.
2. Toss with crushed garlic cloves and olive oil.
3. Sprinkle with rosemary, oregano, tarragon, and basil to taste.
4. Spread in a roasting pan in single layers.
5. Roast approximately 20 minutes at 400°F until veggies are tender and slightly browned, stirring occasionally.
6. Add salt and pepper to taste.
7. Serve immediately while warm.
8. Enjoy!

Personal Notes:

DAY 27

> "Nurturing yourself is not selfish—it's essential
> to your survival and your well-being."
> *—Renee Peterson Trudeau*

WELCOME TO DAY 27. You're about to cross the finish line. But does the thought of eating normally outside of this cleanse make you nervous? Don't be! You've gained so many tools to keep you going strong.

It's a great idea to make a food plan. Document the recipes you enjoyed and map out your meals for the week. Create a shopping list so you can buy everything you need at the grocery store and are completely prepared for each week. Do your best to keep unhealthy, processed foods out of the house. Your family may be reluctant at first, but they will thank you.

In addition to healthy food choices, keep up that water intake as well. It helps the body rid itself of toxins and keeps the bowels running smoothly. Keep putting healthy, nutritious in and let the unhealthy and toxic come out! (Reminder: your weight divided by 2 = amount of daily water in ounces.)

Detox Fact: Water is the most important factor in the body's detoxification process. Remember that in Phase Two of liver detox, you are carrying toxicants out of your body as water-soluble molecules. Staying hydrated keeps your kidneys functioning properly, so they can do their job of transporting waste products into and out of cells and preventing the buildup of blood urea nitrogen, which gets excreted in urine.

LivClear Detox Day 27: Take **two full shakes** today (two scoops each).

Today's Tip: Did you know that cinnamon dates back to ancient Egypt? It was rare, valuable, and regarded as a gift for kings. Why? Cinnamon is a superfood! It has medicinal properties, lowers blood sugar, and prevents amyloid protein buildup in the brain. It contains antioxidants, has anti-inflammatory properties, lowers the risk of heart disease, fights infections, and may even protect against some cancers. Sounds pretty super to us.

Recipe:

Sheet Pan Turkey Dinner

12 ounces green beans, cleaned and trimmed
2 tablespoons olive oil
1 shallot, peeled, halved, and cut into thin slices
salt and pepper
1 lb. sweet potatoes, peeled and cut into small cubes
1 teaspoon salt
⅛ teaspoon cinnamon
24 ounces turkey tenderloin, cut into 4 equal pieces with silver skin trimmed off
2 cloves garlic, minced
1 teaspoon dried rosemary
1 teaspoon dried sage

1. Preheat the oven to 375°F.
2. Arrange green beans evenly on the sheet pan.
3. Drizzle with 1 tablespoon olive oil, add salt, pepper, minced garlic, and shallots. Gently toss to coat.
4. In a medium mixing bowl, toss together the sweet potatoes, 1 tablespoon olive oil, salt, and cinnamon. Arrange sweet potatoes evenly with the green beans on the sheet pan.
5. In the same bowl, add turkey, salt, pepper, rosemary, sage, and remaining garlic. Toss
6. the turkey in the bowl until the seasoning is evenly coating the turkey. Arrange the four pieces into the veggies evenly down the pan.
7. Bake in the oven for 25 minutes or until the turkey juices run clear and an instant-read thermometer reads 165°F when placed in the center.
8. Allow to cool for 5 minutes and serve warm, refrigerate for up to 5 days, or freeze for up to 60 days.
9. Enjoy!

Personal Notes:

DAY 28

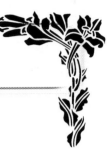

"Embrace and love your body. It's the most
amazing thing you will ever own."
—*Unknown*

WELCOME TO DAY 28—BRAVO! After completing this beautiful
journey, not only do you LOOK different, but you FEEL different, because
YOU are different. The past 28 days have not only given your body the
chance to detox but also to reset. They have also given you an incredible
new lifestyle to follow. Internal organs are operating more efficiently, cell
function is better, and immunity is stronger. These changes may sound
clinical, but the best part is that these changes make you FEEL GREAT!

Are you feeling sad because the journey is over? Perhaps this portion is,
but this only leads you to the next destination, which is the rest of your life.
With the knowledge you've gained, you can easily lead the rest of your life
in good health because you've learned to make better choices.

But none of us are perfect. In the future, if you feel that you've waned
from these good choices, the LivClear Detox is always here for you to come
back to. We all need reminders sometimes. Every once in a while, it's great to
consult this book and refresh your memory and your love for healthy eating.

Detox Fact: Have you heard the term "free radicals" but were never really
sure of what they are? Well, you know they're bad for you, and here's why: A
free radical is defined as "an uncharged molecule (typically highly reactive
and short-lived) having an unpaired valence electron." Huh? They're
basically single atoms that are naturally produced in your body that cause
oxidative stress, which leads to cell damage and a range of diseases. We can
accelerate the production of these atoms with poor lifestyle choices, like
overeating, exposure to pesticides and toxic chemicals, smoking, alcohol,
fried foods, and consuming processed substances (junk food is NOT food,
it's JUNK).

LivClear Detox Day 28: Take **two full shakes** today (two scoops each).

Today's Tip: Your mother always told you to eat your broccoli, and she was absolutely right. Broccoli is a strong source of vitamin C, which is a powerful antioxidant and protects the body from free radicals. Broccoli is the KING of vegetables!

Recipe:

Roasted Salmon with Broccoli

4 salmon fillets
4 cups of broccoli florets (about 2 heads)
3 tablespoons of avocado oil
2 cloves of minced garlic
1½ teaspoon of sea salt
½ teaspoon ground black pepper
1 sliced lemon

1. Preheat the oven to 450°F.
2. Line a baking sheet with parchment paper.
3. Place the fillets on the parchment paper.
4. Drizzle 1 tablespoon of oil over the salmon.
5. Spread the garlic cloves on top.
6. Sprinkle with ½ teaspoon salt and ¼ teaspoon pepper, and place lemon slices on top.
7. Combine florets with 2 tablespoons oil, 1 teaspoon salt, and ¼ teaspoon pepper in a bowl. Evenly coat florets with oil and spices.
8. Arrange broccoli evenly around salmon on baking sheet.
9. Bake 13–15 minutes.
10. Enjoy!

Personal Notes:

YOUR LIVCLEAR DETOX PROGRAM IS COMPLETE: NOW WHAT?

CONGRATULATIONS IN A really BIG way! What you have just completed is so much more than a biotransformation program for supporting the detox pathways in your body. It is the start of an entirely new awareness and lifestyle that you can take with you for the rest of your life. Actually, you can continue to build on the great work that you've done. Yes, you have flooded your body with the necessary nutrients to support the three phases of detoxification, but you have also facilitated healthier cellular function, better energy production, better hormone communication, stronger immunity, keener cognition, deeper sleep, healthier relations, (especially with yourself), increased awareness of healthy choices, broken addictions, and so much more.

Why would you ever want to stop and go back to the life before the LivClear Detoxification Program? You are already building an entirely new lifestyle based on what you have learned over the past 28 days. Let's list some of your victories:

- Completed the goal of the twenty-eight-day LivClear Detoxification Program
- Greater appreciation and understanding of food, its quality, its sources, and its influence on your health
- Better discipline
- Improved sense of self and well-being
- Severed addictions to alcohol, coffee, sugar, wheat, dairy, and other junk
- Severed attachments to unhealthy behaviors
- Created a host of new, healthy behaviors
- Look at food with a different awareness and appreciation
- Demonstrated a commitment to better self-care
- More personal respect and self-appreciation

113

- More respect and admiration from family and friends
- Shift in metabolism
- Weight loss
- Measurable health benefits, including lower cholesterol, decreased blood pressure, lower inflammation, and better sugar regulation
- Reduced risk for heart disease, Alzheimer's, and cancers
- _____ (fill in the blank!)

Here are some guidelines I'd like to share, so that you may continue to benefit from all the great changes and improvements you've made.

Adding foods back in: While there is absolutely nothing wrong with you continuing to adhere to the Basic Dietary Guidelines, there are safe and easy additions you can make. See below on page 118 for a separate guide for introducing suspicious foods back into your diet, with a chart to track changes. Because you have eliminated the most problematic of known antigenic foods and substances, you have reduced immune sensitivity to these. But if you need to avoid any food for an extended period of time, this chart will help you make that determination.

- Reintroduce only one new food at a time. Eat it two to three times in the same day, stop eating it, then wait forty-eight hours to see if you have a reaction. Assess your response over that time, keeping track of your symptoms below. If there is no reaction to a food, you can keep that food in your food plan and continue with the next food for reintroduction. If you are unsure whether you had a reaction, retest the same food in the same manner. (Taken from IFM's Food Reintroduction PDF)
- Eggs, shellfish, and goat milk products are tolerated by most; as is cow's milk that is free of A1 beta-casein. So, I'd suggest starting with these.

When adding a food back into your diet, follow this rule of thumb: Are you in control of the food or substance **OR** is that food or substance in control of you?

- Recall that you have just invested wonderful time, energy, and money into making great changes for yourself. In doing so, you have learned which foods and substances might be triggers for you. I encourage you to avoid anything you know will be a trigger, which can easily pull you right back into unhealthy behaviors
- The question of modification comes up frequently in this discussion. What about alcohol—can I have a glass of wine? What about coffee? Can I go back to enjoying coffee? I really miss it, especially in the morning. Just one cup! Is it OK to have wheat once in a while?
  - Only you can answer these questions honestly for yourself, but I will offer you some insight.
  - Coffee is a wonderful beverage and there are certainly more benefits than harm, as long as you don't abuse it. Dependency is the caution word, as you don't want to have to depend on coffee to boost your energy (wakefulness, yes, but not energy). I actually endorse the bulletproof coffee routine in the morning, as described by Dave Asprey in the Bulletproof Diet. Refer to Day 22 for the recipe to make this delicious and healthy morning beverage.
- If you do choose to use the Bulletproof Coffee recipe, be adamant about using organic, and hopefully mold-free, coffee, and pure coconut or MCT oil. NO sweeteners are allowed or necessary. This morning start helps extend your intermittent fast as well, which has amazing health benefits.
  - Eggs: it may surprise you, but eggs tend to be one of the most poorly tolerated foods. I think, however, it is the commercial versions that come from factory-farmed, drug-laden chickens. If you use eggs, buy them from your local farmer or neighbor where you see the chickens pecking about in the yard.
  - Shellfish: if you're intolerant or sensitive to shellfish like shrimp, clams, mussels etc., you probably already know it, as iodine content in shellfish is a major allergen. However, use the food reintroduction tracker to be sure.
  - Dairy: I'd suggest either A1-free cow's milk or goat-milk-based dairy if you're going to reintroduce this category of foods. Goat

milk is better tolerated by most, so again, pay attention and track your reactions.

- Alcohol: It is toxic and addictive, and though I have found research touting some medicinal benefits of alcohol, other than resveratrol, I am not convinced it is something anyone should consume. At this point, research is about 95 percent against alcohol providing health benefits and only a smidgen suggesting it has health value. The conundrum for me is that we as a species have grown up with alcohol for as long as we have been considered "modern man". Every culture I know has found a way to make some form of tantalizing beverage either through fermentation or distilling. If you choose to consume any alcohol, be sure that you remain in control and know that the distilled versions are better for you than the fermented versions, which are wines and beers.

Twenty-Eight Days And Beyond

It is a myth that it takes only twenty-one days to create a new habit and undo an old one. I mentioned earlier, way back in the introduction section, that research suggests it takes an average of sixty-six days. Regardless of your age, whether twenty-five or sixty-five years, do you think that you've undone a lifetime of unhealthy habits in four weeks? Maybe, but you would be one of the fortunate few, as most of us mere mortals need a bit more practice with undoing and new learning. That is what you will want to do now: continue learning about yourself and how you came to be who you are. How did you learn to make the choices you've made? How did you come to believe what you think is true or not? Because, I promise you, it is the belief system you learned in your first seven years of life on this planet that controls 95 percent of your behaviors.

By choosing to participate in this detoxification program, you've initiated an incredible shift in your self-awareness. Everything in your life right now looks and feels different. I encourage you to continue exploring the proverbial "whys" of who you are, how you got here, and how to move forward. These are the ancient perennial questions we all must satisfy. You have just entered on the path of your own journey.

In closing, I'd like you to know how much you're appreciated. Even though I may not know you, in a great way, I do. I know that you are interested in making this world a healthier, more vibrant, and a more enjoyable place to live. I know that love and kindness mean much to you. I know that you have respect for yourself, for others, and this planet. I know that you have love in your being, and that you have allowed it to shine forth from the inner sanctum of your being. And for that I am truly grateful. May your light and love continue to shine and brighten our world.

Food Reintroduction
- Symptoms Tracker-

Reintroduce only one new food at a time. Eat it 2-3 times in the same day, stop eating it, then wait 48 hours to see if you have a reaction. Assess your response over that time, keeping track of your symptoms below. If there is no reaction to a food, you can keep that food in your food plan and continue with the next food for reintroduction. If you are unsure whether you had a reaction, retest the same food in the same manner. If you require more space, copy the blank chart for a second page.

	Day 1	Day 2	Day 3	Day 4
Time				
Food				
Digestion/Bowel Function				
Joint/Muscle Aches				
Headache/ Pressure				
Nasal or Chest Congestion				
Kidney/Bladder Function				
Skin				
Energy Level				

To Contact Dr. Bump or
to Order the LivClear
Program please call:
973-827-3500
Or
www.drbump.com

DR. BUMP'S RECIPES

TABLE OF CONTENTS

DR. BUMP'S RECIPES

Please Note: All recipes are
"Gut Rehab and Dysbiosis" Friendly.
*** indicates Not Detox Friendly.

DR. BUMP'S BREAKFAST RECIPES

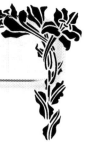

ASPARAGUS WITH POACHED EGG ***

Not detox friendly- contains egg

32 spears asparagus, (or 1 bunch)   1 lemon, juiced and zested
1 Tbs olive oil   4 eggs
3 cloves of garlic, minced   salt and pepper

Procedure

1. Bring a large pot of water to a boil.
2. Separately, heat the oil in a large sauté pan on medium heat. Add the minced garlic, lemon juice and zest and asparagus spears. Sauté and use tongs to move the asparagus around until they are cooked through, approximately 3-5 minutes.
3. Once the pot of water has come to a boil, reduce the heat to low and ensure that no bubbles are breaking the surface. Crack each egg into a ramekin, then gently add to the pot of water. Cook each egg for 3 minutes. Then remove the egg with a slotted spoon and dab the excess water on a paper towel.
4. To assemble, add a few asparagus spears to a plate, top with a poached egg, season with salt and pepper Servings: 4

Preparation Time: 5 minutes
Cooking Time: 15 minutes
Total Time: 20 minutes

Source
Author: Lisa Bryan

AVOCADO EGG BOATS ***

This recipe modified from the original. Not detox diet friendly- contains egg

2 ripe avocados, halved and pitted
4 large eggs
Kosher salt
Freshly ground black pepper
Freshly chopped chives, for garnish

Procedure

1. Preheat oven to 350°. Scoop about 1 tablespoon worth of avocado out of each half; discard or reserve for another use.
2. Place hollowed avocados in a baking dish, then crack eggs into a bowl, one at a time. Using a spoon, transfer one yolk to each avocado half, then spoon in as much egg white as you can fit without spilling over.
3. Season with salt and pepper and bake until whites are set and yolks are no longer runny, 20 to 25 minutes. (Cover with foil if avocados are beginning to brown.)
4. Top avocados with chives before serving.

Servings: 4

Preparation Time: 10 minutes
Total Time: 40 minutes

Source
Author: LINDSAY FUNSTON
Source: Delish

BRUSSEL SPROUTS HASH ***

This recipe is not detox friendly- it contains egg. You can make detox friendly by omitting the egg.

6 slices uncured sugar free bacon, cut into 1" pieces
1/2 onion, chopped
1 lb brussel sprouts, trimmed and quartered

Kosher salt
Freshly ground black pepper
1/4 tsp crushed red pepper flakes
2 cloves garlic, minced
4 large eggs

Procedure

1. In a large skillet over medium heat, cook bacon until crispy. Turn off heat and transfer bacon to a paper towel lined plate. Drain all but about 1 tablespoon bacon fat.
2. Turn heat back to medium and add onion and brussel sprouts to the skillet. Cook, stirring occasionally, until vegetables begin to soften and turn golden. Season with salt, pepper, and red pepper flakes.
3. Add 2 tablespoons of water and cover skillet. Cook until brussel sprouts are tender and water has evaporated, about 5 minutes. (If all the water evaporates before the brussel sprouts are tender, add more water to skillet and cover for a couple minutes more.) Add garlic to skillet and cook until fragrant, 1 minute.
4. Using a wooden spoon, make four holes in the hash to reveal bottom of skillet. Crack an egg into each hole and season each egg with salt and pepper. Replace lid and cook until eggs are cooked to your liking, about 5 minutes for a just runny egg.
5. Sprinkle cooked bacon bits over entire skillet and serve warm.

Servings: 4

Preparation Time: 10 minutes
Total Time: 40 minutes

Source
Author: LENA ABRAHAM
Source: Delish

HEALTHY BREAKFAST CASSEROLE ***

This recipe is not Detox diet friendly- it contains eggs

16 large eggs, beaten
1 1/2 lb ground turkey
2 Tbs avocado oil
1/2 onion, diced
1 green bell pepper, diced
2 green onion, finely sliced
14 oz can artichoke hearts, chopped

2 cups packed fresh baby spinach, plus extra for the top
1 tsp chili powder
1/2 tsp cumin
1/2 tsp oregano
salt and pepper

Procedure

1. Preheat your oven to 375 degrees
2. Heat the oil in a sauté pan on medium heat. Add the onion and bell pepper and give it a quick stir. Add the ground turkey and use a large spoon to break up the turkey.
3. Add the spices, salt and pepper and stir to combine everything. Cook for approximately 10 minutes, or until there's no liquid in the pan and the meat is cooked through and browned.
4. Add the spinach to the meat mixture and stir for 1-2 minutes or until the spinach just starts to wilt.
5. Transfer the meat to a 9x13-inch casserole dish and evenly cover the bottom. Top with the artichoke hearts and beaten eggs.
6. Sprinkle the green onion and a handful of spinach on top.
7. Cook the casserole in the oven for 40-45 minutes, or until cooked through.

Servings: 12

Total Time: 1 hour and 5 minutes

Source
Author: Lisa Bryan
Source: Downshiftology

LIVCLEAR SHAKE IDEAS

GREENS
spinach, chard or baby kale

VEGETABLES
cucumber, carrot, cauliflower, zucchini (be creative)

FRUIT
blueberries or strawberries fresh or frozen (be careful fruit adds sugar)

FATS
avocado, cashews or almonds in nut or sugar free nut butter form

LIQUID
almond or coconut milk, coconut water, brewed herbal flavored tea or plain water
add a few ice cubes for a chilled drink

2 SCOOPS LIVCLEAR POWDER
SPICES
cinnamon, ginger, nutmeg, allspice, cardamom add a dash
vanilla, peppermint sugar free extract

Procedure

1. add your desired variety of ingredients to a Vitamix type blender
   and sip- mindfully

PALEO AND WHOLE30 GROUND TURKEY HASH ***

Omit fried egg on top for detox friendly recipe.

2 Tbs avocado oil, divided	4 eggs
1 sweet onion, diced to 1/2" cube	1 zucchini, diced to 1/2" cube
2 cloves garlic, minced	1 yellow squash, diced to 1/2" cube
1 lb ground turkey	1 bell pepper, diced to 1/2" cube
1/2 tsp dried thyme	1 Tbs fresh parsley, chopped
1/4 tsp dried oregano	sea salt, to taste
1/4 tsp red pepper flakes	cracked black pepper, to taste

Procedure

1. Heat a 12" skillet over medium high heat. Add 1 Tbsp avocado oil and heat until shimmering. Add the onion and saute, stirring frequently, until the onions are soft, 4-5 minutes. Add the garlic and saute until fragrant, 1 minute.
2. Add the turkey to the onions and garlic, along with the herbs, red pepper flakes, and salt and pepper to taste. Saute, stirring frequently to break up the meat, until the turkey is no longer pink, 5-7 minutes.
3. Push the turkey/onion mixture to the edges of the pan and add 1 tsp oil to the center of the pan. Add the zucchini and squash to the oil, and saute, stirring frequently, until the squash is tender but still retains a bite, about 5 minutes. Add the bell pepper to the pan and stir to combine all ingredients. Continue to saute the hash, stirring frequently, for an additional 3-4 minutes, or until the bell pepper is just barely cooked.
4. Taste for seasoning and add additional salt and pepper if needed. Divide the hash between 4 plates and sprinkle with fresh parsley.
5. Wipe out the pan, add the last two tsp avocado oil, and heat until shimmering. Crack four eggs into the pan, one at a time, and fry until the whites are set, 3-4 minutes. Top each plate of hash with a fried egg and serve immediately.

Servings: 4

Preparation Time: 5 minutes
Cooking Time: 25 minutes
Total Time: 30 minutes

Recipe Tips

For a meal prep version, divide the turkey hash into four single serving containers and store in the fridge for up to 5 days. When you're ready to eat, reheat on high for 1 minute, and top with a freshly fried egg.

Source
Author: Danielle Esposti
Source: Our Salty Kitchen

SPEEDY SHANGHAI STIR-FRY

1 lb ground pork
1/4 tsp sea salt
6 cups shredded green cabbage (about 1 pound). I used a food processor to shred cabbage.
1 Tbs coconut oil

STIR-FRY SAUCE:

1/4 cup coconut aminos
1 Tbs fresh lime juice
1 tsp ginger powder
1 tsp rice syrup

1/2 tsp garlic powder
1/2 tsp arrowroot
Green onions

Procedure

1. In a large, deep skillet or wok (use my extra large skillet), cook the ground pork over medium heat until no longer pink. Season with salt and transfer to a fine-mesh strainer set over the sink to drain. Wipe the skillet clean.
2. In the same skillet, saute the cabbage in coconut oil over medium-high heat until wilted but still crunchy. 6-7 minutes.
3. In a small bow, whisk together the ingredients for the sauce.
4. Return the pork to the pan and combine well with the cabbage. Add the sauce and continuously toss the pork with the cabbage until the sauce has thickened slightly and the cabbage is translucent, 1-2 minutes. Serve immediately with green onions.

Servings: 4

Source
Author: Aleana Haber and Sarah Ballantyne
Source: The Healing Kitchen

DR. BUMP'S CONDIMENTS AND DRESSINGS RECIPES

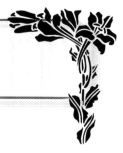

AVOCADO MAYO

2 large avocado, peeled and pitted
6 Tbsp olive oil
2 Tbsp fresh lemon juice
1/2 tsp fine sea salt
1/4 tsp garlic powder

Procedure

1. Place the pitted and peeled avocados in a blender. with the blender running, slowly drizzle the olive oil to combine the avocados with the oil.
2. Add the remaining ingredients and puree until smooth.

Yield: 1 cup

Preparation Time: 5 minutes
Total Time: 5 minutes

Source
Source: The Healing Kitchen

CAESAR DRESSING

1/2 cup coconut cream or full fat coconut milk
1/2 cup mashed avocado
1/4 cup olive oil
2 cloves garlic, pressed
1 Tbs lemon juice, freshly squeezed

2 tsp mashed anchovies
1/2 tsp fish sauce (a clean brand like Red Boat)
1/2 tsp fine sea salt
1/4 tsp garlic powder
1/4 tsp onion powder

Procedure

1. Place all ingredients in a blender & blend on high speed until smooth.

Yield: 1 cup

Preparation Time: 8 minutes
Total Time: 8 minutes

Source
Author: The Healing Kitchen

CAULI'FREDO SAUCE

Serve over chicken, seared shrimp or toss with broccoli

2 cups cauliflower florets - about 1/2 a head
1 Tbsp minced garlic divided
1 Tbsp olive oil
1/2 tsp fine sea salt
1/4 cup chicken broth

Procedure

1. Steam cauliflower in a lidded steamer basket set over a pot of boiling water for 4-5 minutes, until tender. Drain and transfer to blender.
2. Meanwhile, in a small skillet over medium heat, cook the garlic in the olive oil for 2-3 minutes, until fragrant, making sure that the garlic does not burn.
3. Spoon the garlic into the blender, add the salt and chicken broth and puree on high speed until smooth. For a thinner sauce, add more broth or water 2 Tablespoons at a time until the desired thickness in reached.

Yield: 1 cup

Preparation Time: 5 minutes
Cooking Time: 8 minutes
Total Time: 13 minutes

Source
Source: The Healing Kitchen

CREAMY DILL DRESSING

Juice of 2 Lemons
1 clove of Garlic
3/4 cup Dill, packed
3/4 cup Olive Oil
1/2 cup Sunflower Seeds, soaked
Sea Salt and Pepper to taste

Procedure

1. Blend all ingredients, except oil, in blender. Slowly adding in olive oil. Blend until creamy. Source

Author: unknown

GARLIC- DILL RANCH DRESSING

1/4 cup coconut cream, chilled
1/3 cup coconut oil
6 Tbsp olive oil
1 Tbsp lemon juice, freshly squeezed
1 Tbsp minced yellow onion
1-1/2 tsp dried chives

1 tsp minced garlic
1 tsp fresh dill minced
1/2 tsp dried parsley
1/4 tsp garlic powder
1/4 tsp onion powder

Procedure

1. In a mixing bowl, combine the coconut cream, coconut oil, olive oil and lemon juice.
2. Beat with hand mixer on medium speed until smooth and creamy. At this point you have a basic Mayonnaise that can be used in cold sauces, salad dressings and salads.
3. Add the remaining ingredients and mix with a spoon until well combined

Yield: 1 1/4 cup

Preparation Time: 10 minutes
Total Time: 10 minutes

Source
Source: The Healing Kitchen Cookbook

GREEK DRESSING

1/2 cup Olive Oil
1/3 cup Lemon Juice
2 Tbs Mint, minced
2 cloves Garlic, mashed and minced
1/4 tsp Paprika,
Sea Salt and Pepper to taste

Procedure

1. Whisk everything together in a bowl. Let sit for at least one hour.
2. Store in a glass jar, shake before using.

Source
Author: unknown

LEMON TAHINI DRESSING

1/2 cup Olive Oil
1/4 cup Sesame Seeds or Tahini
1/2 – 2/3 cup Lemon Juice
1 Clove Garlic
Sea salt and pepper to taste

Procedure

1. Blend all ingredients in a blender, until creamy.
2. Try dressing on wraps or as a dip

Source Author: unknown

SMOKY ARTICHOKE BABA GHANOUSH

Serve with roast chicken or with vegetables as a dip.

1 14 oz can artichoke hearts, drained
1/4 cup olive oil
1-1/2 Tbsp fresh lemon juice
2 large cloves garlic
3/4 tsp smoked sea salt

Procedure

1. Place all of the ingredients in a blender or food processor and pulse until smooth about, 1 minute

Yield: 1 cup

Preparation Time: 7 minutes
Total Time: 7 minutes

Source
Source: The Healing Kitchen Cook book

STRAWBERY LIME DRESSING

1/2 cup strawberries
1/4 cup olive oil
1 tbs lime juice fresh
1 tbs coconut aminos
1/2 tsp fine sea
salt 1/4 tsp powdered ginger

Procedure

1. Remove the green tops form the strawberries. Place all ingredients in a blender and blend on high speed until very smooth.

Yield: 1 cup

Preparation Time: 8 minutes
Total Time: 8 minutes

Source
Author: The Healing Kitchen

TZATZIKI SAUCE

Use as a salad dressing or dip for vegetables

1 1/2 cups peeled, seeded and chopped cucumber
1/2 cup coconut cream, chilled
1/2 cup mashed avocado
2 Tbsp fresh lemon juice
2 Tbsp chopped fresh dill
1 clove garlic, chopped
1/2 tsp fine sea salt

Procedure

1. Place all of the ingredients in a food processor or blender and blend on high speed until smooth.

Yield: 1 cup

Preparation Time: 10 minutes
Total Time: 10 minutes

Source
Source: The Healing Kitchen cook book

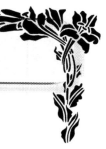

DR. BUMP'S DINNER RECIPES

BROILED SALMON

4 (4-oz.) salmon fillets
1 Tbs Grainy mustard
2 cloves garlic, finely minced
1 Tbs finely minced shallots
2 tsp fresh thyme leaves, chopped, plus more for garnish
2 tsp fresh rosemary, chopped
Juice of 1/2 lemon
Salt
Freshly ground black pepper Lemon slices, for serving

Procedure

1. Heat broiler and line a baking sheet with parchment. In a small bowl, mix together mustard, garlic, shallot, thyme, rosemary, and lemon juice and season with salt and pepper. Spread mixture all over salmon fillets and broil, 7 to 8 minutes.
2. Garnish with more thyme and lemon slices and serve.

Servings: 4

Preparation Time: 15 minutes
Total Time: 15 minutes

Source
Author: Delish

CARAMELIZED ONION & HERB MEATLOAF

1 pound ground beef

1 pound ground pork

1 Tbsp dried thyme leaves, crushed

1 1/2 tsp dried rubbed sage

1 tsp sea salt

3/4 cup caramelized onion (see how to make below)

2 Tbsp water for topping

1 Tbsp olive oil

2 whole Vidalia onion

Procedure

1. oven to 375 degrees
2. Grease 9 x 5 inch loaf pan.
3. In large mixing bowl use your hands to combine the beef, pork, thyme, sage and 1 tsp of the salt
4. To carmalize onions heat 1 Tablespoon olive oil & add 2 sliced Vidalia onions, cook covered over medium heat for 20 minutes. stirring the onions and browned bits from the bottom of the pan every 5 minutes until golden and tender
5. Add 3/4 cup caramelized onions and mix.
6. Transfer to prepared loaf pan
7. Bake for 40 to 45 minutes until the meat has pulled away from the sides of the pan and the internal temperature has reached 150 degrees. Do not over cook or the meatloaf will dry out
8. Meanwhile, place the remaining caramelized onions, 1/4 tsp salt and water in a blender and pulse until chunky puree forms.
9. Top the cooked meatloaf with the onion puree and broil on high for 5 minutes until the onions are deep golden brown.
10. Let rest for 10 minutes to let the juices reabsorb before slicing

Servings: 6

Preparation Time: 5 minutes

Cooking Time: 50 minutes

Total Time: 55 minutes

CAULIFLOWER ARROZ CON POLLO

2 lbs bone in skin on chicken thighs
3 Tbs avocado oil, divided
1 tsp sea salt, divided
1/2 tsp black pepper
1 large yellow onion, diced
2 cloves garlic, minced
3 cups cauliflower rice
1/4 cup canned diced tomatoes

1/4 cup chicken broth
1/2 cup green peas
1 1/2 tsp turmeric powder
1 tsp cumin
2 tsp dried oregano
2 Tbs fresh cilantro, chopped
2 limes, quartered

Procedure

1. Pat the chicken dry and lightly season with salt and pepper.
2. Using a large skillet, heat about 2 tbsp of oil in the pan. Once the oil is hot, add the chicken. Sear for about 3-4 minutes on each side or until lightly crisp. The internal temperature should read 165 F. Set aside on a plate.
3. Add more oil if necessary, and saute the onion and garlic until the onion is translucent and the garlic is fragrant.
4. Stir in the cauliflower rice and gently saute for 2-3 minutes. Stir in the diced tomato, broth, peas, and season with turmeric, cumin and cilantro. Stir well to combine and bring to the liquid to a low simmer.
5. Add the chicken back to the pan and evenly disperse. Cover the pot and allow to simmer for 5-8 minutes or until the liquid has reduced and the chicken is heated through.
6. Serve topped with chopped cilantro and limes.

Servings: 4

Preparation Time: 10 minutes
Cooking Time: 25 minutes
Total Time: 35 minutes

Source
Author: MICHELLE
Source: Unbound Wellness

COCONUT CHICKEN CURRY WITH CASHEWS

2 lbs skinless boneless chicken thighs, cut in 3-inch chunks
Salt and pepper
1 Tbs grated ginger
2 tsp grated garlic
¼ tsp cloves
¼ tsp fennel seeds
¼ tsp cardamom seeds
¼ tsp allspice berries
¼ tsp cumin seeds
¼ tsp coriander seeds
¼ tsp turmeric
¼ tsp cayenne, or more to taste
3 Tbs lemon juice

¾ cup raw cashews
¼ cup shredded dried unsweetened coconut
1 lb small parsnips, peeled and cut in 2-inch batons
2 Tbs ghee, coconut oil or vegetable oil
1 ½ cups finely diced onion
1 Tbs tomato paste
1 2-inch piece cinnamon stick
3 cups chicken broth or water
1 cup thick coconut milk
A few sprigs mint and cilantro for garnish, optional

Procedure

1. Season chicken generously with salt and pepper and put it in a mixing bowl. Add ginger and garlic and massage into meat. In a dry skillet over medium heat, toast cloves, fennel, cardamom, allspice, cumin and coriander until fragrant, about 2 minutes. Grind the toasted spices to a fine powder in an electric spice mill and add to chicken. Add turmeric, cayenne and lemon juice and mix well. Let marinate at room temperature for at least 15 minutes, or refrigerate up to 1 hour.

2. Heat oven to 375 degrees. Put cashews on a baking sheet and roast until lightly browned, 8 to 10 minutes. Remove and set aside to cool. Spread the shredded coconut on the baking sheet and toast until lightly browned, about 5 minutes, then let cool. Grind the coconut with 1/4 cup cashews in a spice mill or small food processor to make a rough powder. Reserve 1/2 cup roasted cashews for garnish.

3. Bring a small saucepan of lightly salted water to a simmer, then add parsnips and cook until tender, about 10 minutes. Drain and cool.

4. In a wide heavy-bottomed pot, heat ghee over medium-high heat. Add cooked parsnips, and sauté until lightly browned. Remove and

reserve. Add chicken pieces to the pot, stirring occasionally until lightly browned, about 5 minutes, then remove and set aside. Add onions and cook until softened, about 5 minutes more. Add tomato paste and let it sizzle with onions for a minute or two. Add broth and bring to a brisk simmer, stirring with a wooden spoon and scraping up any caramelized bits from the pot. Add cinnamon stick, chicken and the ground coconut and cashew mixture. Adjust heat to a gentle simmer, cover and cook for about 30 minutes, until chicken is tender. Taste the sauce and adjust seasoning if necessary.

5. To finish the dish, stir in coconut milk and add reserved parsnips. Cook for 3 to 4 minutes, until parsnips are heated through and the sauce has thickened slightly. Transfer to a serving bowl and sprinkle with reserved cashews. Garnish with mint and cilantro sprigs, if using.

Servings: 4

Total Time: 1 hour

Source
Author: David Tanis

DON'T FEEL LIKE COOKING A FULL RECIPE?

Author Notes

COOK UP AN ORGANIC PROTEIN: PAN FRY, ROAST OR BRAISE
Beef- ground, steak, roast, cubed
Chicken-ground, breast, thighs, whole
Lamb-Ground, cubes, roast
Pork-Ground, tenderloin, chops, roast
Turkey-Ground, breast, leg, whole
Fish, Shrimp, Scallop-wild caught

VEGETABLES- ORGANIC
Cook- Steam, roast, pressure cook or pan sauté
Eat raw- salad, or cut up & added to plate
You can always make a big batch and grab as you need during the week, or freeze to use later.

EASY INSTANT POT SHREDDED BEEF

2 Tbs avocado oil
2 lbs chuck roast, sliced into cubes (or sub beef stew meat)
1 tsp sea salt
1/3 tsp black pepper
2 cloves garlic, minced
2 tsp onion powder
2 bay leaves
1 cup beef broth
Juice of one lime

Procedure

1. Add the avocado oil to the instant pot and set to saute. Once the oil is hot, add the beef and season with salt and pepper. Saute for 2-3 minutes on each side to very lightly brown. Hit cancel on the instant pot.
2. Add the remainder of the ingredients to the instant pot.
3. Place the lid on the instant pot with pressure valve sealed. Hit "Manual" and cook on high pressure for 90 minutes.
4. Let the instant pot to come to pressure, cook, and let the pressure release naturally. When the pressure is released, remove the lid from the instant pot.
5. Remove the bay leaves and carefully shred the meat with two forks. Use the meat as all-purpose meat in a variety of recipes and top with herbs or lime juice if desired.

Servings: 8

Preparation Time: 5 minutes
Cooking Time: 1 hour and 30 minutes
Total Time: 1 hour and 35 minutes

Source
Author: MICHELLE
Source: Unbound Wellness

GARLIC BUTTER GROUND TURKEY WITH CAULIFLOWER

1 lb ground turkey (or ground chicken)

1/2 head cauliflower, sliced into florets and steamed

2 Tbs vegetable oil

1 Tbs lemon juice

3 Tbs butter

2 Tbs minced garlic

1 Tbs onion powder

1/4 cup coconut amino

2 tsp sesame oil

Fresh chopped cilantro (or parsley)

1/4 cup water

Red chili pepper flakes

Lemon slices, for garnish

Procedure

1. To make the Garlic Butter Turkey with Cauliflower: Heat a large skillet over medium-low with one tablespoon vegetable oil. Saute the pre-cooked cauliflower florets in the skillet, until slightly golden brown – make sure not to burn cauliflower. Deglaze with lemon juice, add in some fresh cilantro, salt and pepper to your taste, and toss to coat well. Remove to a shallow plate.

2. In the same skillet (rinse the skillet if cauliflower has burnt), melt butter with one tablespoon oil and cook ground turkey, breaking the meat apart with a wooden spoon. When the turkey meat is no longer pink, add garlic, the onion powder and give a quick stir. Add coconut aminos. water and continue cooking, stirring regularly, for a couple of minutes.

3. Push ground turkey aside and return the cauliflower to the skillet. Reheat quickly and coat cauliflower in the sauce. Add a drizzle of sesame oil, sprinkle with fresh chopped cilantro, red chili pepper flakes and garnish with lemon slices. Serve the Garlic Butter Turkey with Cauliflower immediately – enjoy!

Servings: 4

GARLICKY GREEK CHICKEN

3 Tbs extra-virgin olive oil, divided Juice of 1 lemon
3 cloves garlic, minced
1 tsp dried oregano
1 lb chicken thighs salt
Freshly ground black pepper
1/2 lb asparagus, ends removed
1 zucchini, sliced into half moons
1 lemon, sliced

Procedure

1. In a large bowl, combine 2 tablespoons olive oil, lemon juice, garlic, and oregano. Whisk until combined then add chicken thighs and toss to coat. Cover bowl with plastic wrap and let marinate in the refrigerator for at least 15 minutes and up to 2 hours.
2. When you're ready to cook the chicken, preheat oven to 425°. In a large ovenproof skillet over medium-high heat, heat remaining tablespoon olive oil. Season both sides of marinated chicken with salt and pepper, then add chicken skin-side down and pour in the remaining marinade.
3. Sear until the skin becomes golden and crispy, about 10 minutes. Flip chicken and add asparagus, zucchini and lemons to the skillet.
4. Transfer pan to oven and cook until the chicken is cooked through and the vegetables are tender, about 15 minutes.

Servings: 4
Yield: 4

Preparation Time: 20 minutes
Cooking Time: 30 minutes
Total Time: 50 minutes

Source
Author: LAUREN MIYASHIRO
Source: Delish

GREEK MEATBALLS WITH AVOCADO TZATZIKI SAUCE

FOR THE GREEK MEATBALLS:

1 lb ground lamb (or ground beef)
½ medium red onion, finely diced (about ½ cup)
2 cloves garlic, minced
zest of ½ lemon
1 dried oregano
1 tsp ground coriander
½ tsp ground cumin
sea salt and pepper, to taste

1 avocado
1 small/medium cucumber or ½ large cucumber, cut in half and seeds scraped out with a spoon
2 cloves garlic
1 Tbs red onion, diced
juice of 1 lemon
1 Tbs fresh dill (or mint, depending on your preference)
¼ cup goat yogurt
sea salt and pepper, to taste

Procedure

1. Preheat oven to 350 degrees F.
2. Combine all the meatball ingredients together and form into approximately 1-1/2 to 2 inch balls.
3. Place on a raised edge baking pan and bake for 25 minutes.
4. To make Avocado Tzatziki Sauce:
5. Combine all avocado tzatziki sauce ingredients together in a food processor or blender.
6. Blend until smooth and creamy.
7. Serve with avocado tzatziki sauce and enjoy!

Yield: 25-30 Greek meatballs

Source
Author: Kelly from Primally Inspired

GRILLED LEMON BUTTER SALMON

4 Tbs butter melted 2 cloves garlic, minced
1 tsp lemon zest
1 tsp kosher salt
Pinch red pepper flakes
4 (6-oz.) salmon fillets
6 lemons, sliced
Freshly chopped parsley, for serving

Procedure

1. Stir butter, garlic, lemon zest, salt, and red pepper flakes to combine. Spoon mixture all over salmon fillets.
2. Preheat grill to medium-high. Arrange lemons on grill and place salmon fillets on top. Cover grill and cook until salmon is cooked through and flakes easily with a fork, 15 to 20 minutes. (Exact cooking time will vary based on the thickness of your fillets.)
3. Serve with grilled lemon slices and garnish with parsley, if using.

Yield: 4 SERVINGS

Preparation Time: 5 minutes
Total Time: 25 minutes

Source
Author: LAUREN MIYASHIRO
Source: Delish

GROUND BEEF TACO BOWL

FOR THE CAULIFLOWER RICE:

1 head cauliflower
1 Tbs avocado oil or olive oil
1 tsp garlic powder
1 tsp onion powder
1 tsp cilantro
1/2 lime, juiced

FOR THE TACO MEAT:

2 tsp avocado oil or olive oil
1 lb ground beef
1/2 Tbs chili powder
1/2 tsp onion powder
1 tsp garlic powder
1/2 tsp red pepper flakes
1 tsp cumin
1/2 tsp paprika
1 tsp oregano
1/4 cup water

1/2 cup tomato sauce topping ideas:
red onion
sliced radishes
avocado
lime juice
jalapenos
tomatoes
mixed greens
cilantro

Procedure

1. for the cauliflower rice:
2. Chop the cauliflower into large chunks and place them in a food processor. (Work in two separate batches if you are doing a whole head of cauliflower.) Pulse until the cauliflower has the texture of rice.
3. In a large skillet, heat avocado oil over medium heat. Place the cauliflower rice in the skillet and saute for about 3-5 minutes. Season with garlic powder, onion powder, salt, and lime juice. Transfer the cauliflower rice into a large bowl. Set aside.
4. for the taco meat:
5. In the same skillet, heat oil over medium-high heat. Add the ground beef to the skillet and using a spatula, break the beef into smaller pieces. Cook the ground beef until no longer pink. Add water,

tomato sauce, and spices to the ground beef. Stir together and bring to a simmer. Simmer for 3-5 minutes or until little liquid remains in the skillet.

6. Make the taco bowl by adding the cauliflower rice to the bottom, and then adding the taco meat. Add the toppings of your choice and garnish with cilantro and lime juice.

Servings: 4

Preparation Time: 10 minutes
Cooking Time: 15 minutes
Total Time: 25 minutes

Source
Author: Abbey Blackwell
Source: Healthy consultant

INSTANT POT CHICKEN NO-TORTILLA SOUP

2 Tbs avocado oil
1 onion, diced
1 jalapeno, diced and seeded
3 cloves garlic, minced
2 medium zucchinis, chopped
(about 2 cups)
4 cups chicken broth
1 15 oz can fire roasted tomatoes

Juice of one lime
1 tsp sea salt
1/2 tsp black pepper
1 tsp cumin
2 tsp oregano
1 lb chicken breast
2 Tbs cilantro
1-2 mediun avocados, sliced

Procedure

1. Set the instant pot to saute and add the avocado oil. Once heated, add the onion, jalapeno and garlic. Cook for 3-4 minutes or until the onion is slightly translucent.
2. Add the zucchini and saute for another 1-2 minutes to soften.
3. Pour in the broth, tomato, lime juice, chicken, and seasonings (reserving cilantro to serve) and stir well to combine.
4. Hit "cancel" on the instant pot and place on the lid with the valve sealed. Set the instant pot to high pressure for 12 minutes.
5. Allow to come to pressure and cook. Quick release the pressure and carefully remove the lid. Use a meat thermometer to ensure the chicken is 165F. Set the instant pot to saute for longer if needed. Pull the chicken out and shred with two forks. Add back to the soup and stir.
6. Serve topped with cilantro, avocado, and additional lime juice to taste.

Servings: 4

Preparation Time: 10 minutes
Cooking Time: 20 minutes

Source
Author: MICHELLE
Source: Unbound Wellness

Author Notes

To make in the slow cooker, add all of the ingredients to the slow cooker and set to low for 6-8 hours. Remove the chicken and shred when cooked through. Serve topped with cilantro and avocado.

KENYAN BRAISED COLLARD GREENS AND GROUND BEEF

1 tsp olive oil
1/2 white onion, coarsely chopped
2 cloves garlic, chopped
1 jalapeno, seeded and chopped
1 lb 90% lean ground beef
1/2 tsp black pepper
1/2 tsp ground cinnamon
1/2 tsp ground ginger
1/2 tsp turmeric

1 tsp salt
1 tsp ground cumin
1 tsp ground coriander
1 bunch, 8 leaves collard greens, stems removed sliced into 1-inch srips
15 grape tomatoes, quartered
1 tsp lemon juice

Procedure

1. Warm the olive oil in a large skillet over medium heat.
2. Add the onion and saute until soft, about 4 minutes.
3. Add the garlic and jalapeño and saute until fragrant, about 1 minute.
4. Add the ground beef and seasonings and cook until browned, about 6 to 8 minutes.
5. Add the collard greens and tomatoes and saute until wilted, about 4 minutes.
6. Stir everything gently as it cooks, careful not to mush the tomatoes.
7. Add the lemon juice, season with salt and pepper to taste and serve.

Servings: 4

Preparation Time: 15 minutes
Cooking Time: 15 minutes
Total Time: 30 minutes

Source
Author: https://www.skinnytaste.com

KETO CREAMY CHICKEN AND EGGPLANT CASSEROLE

4 Tbs coconut oil, to cook with 3 chicken breasts diced
1 eggplant cubed
4 cloves of garlic, minced
8 cherry tomatoes, diced small
2 cups of spinach chopped
2 Tbs of Italian seasoning
1/4 cup of fresh parsley, chopped
1 can of coconut milk
Salt and pepper, to taste

Procedure

1. Preheat oven to 400 F
2. In a large pan, melt the coconut oil over medium-high heat. Add the chicken, eggplant, garlic, cherry tomatoes, and spinach. Sauté until the chicken is cooked and the vegetables are soft.
3. Add the Italian seasoning, parsley, coconut milk, and season with salt and pepper to taste.
4. Pour mixture into a greased baking dish and bake for 20 minutes.

Servings: 4

Preparation Time: 15 minutes
Cooking Time: 20 minutes
Total Time: 35 minutes

Source
Source: ketosummit

KUNG PAO CHICKEN ZUCCHINI NOODLES

1 medium onion, 1/2" dice

1 red bell pepper, 1/2" dice

4 large carrots, thinly sliced

4 medium zucchini

1 Tbs minced fresh ginger

4 cloves garlic, minced

2 tsp red pepper flakes

1 pkg boneless skinless chicken breast or 4 thighs, cut into 1/2" pieces

1/4 cup avocado oil- divided

1/4 cup coconut aminos

2 TBS rice syrup

2 Tbs lime juice

4–6 drops (less than 1/4 teaspoon) toasted sesame oil

1 Tbs tapioca starch

GARNISHES:

1 cup toasted cashews

1/2 cup thinly sliced green onions

Procedure

1. Prepare the onion, bell pepper, and carrots and set aside in a bowl.
2. Spiralize the zucchini and set the noodles aside in a bowl.
3. Place the ginger, garlic, and red pepper flakes in a small bowl and set aside.
4. Mix together all the ingredients for the sauce, coconut aminos, lime juice, rice syrup, sesame oil, tapioca starch and 2 TBS avocado oil making sure there are no lumps of tapioca starch.
5. Preheat a large (6 quart) stainless steel fry pan over high heat. When the pan is hot, add 2 Tablespoons of the avocado oil and the cubed chicken to the pan. Stir fry for a couple of minutes turning twice, waiting for browned edges appear before turning. When the chicken is mostly done, remove it from the pan and set aside until the end.
6. Add the remaining oil to the pan along with the onions, bell pepper, and carrots. If there's a lot of browned bits on the bottom add 2 tablespoons of water as well and scrape it off as you stir fry the vegetables. When they're crisp tender, add the ginger, garlic, and red pepper flakes. Stir fry until fragrant, about 1 minute. Then add the chicken back into the pan along with the zucchini noodles and

sauce. Stir fry for 1-2 minutes scraping the bottom with a metal spatula as you go. Remove the pan from the heat when the zucchini noodles still look underdone and bit firm, they will soften in the next few minutes without further cooking. Season to taste with sea salt if desired.

7. Serve immediately with the toasted cashews and green onions.

Yield: 4-6 servings

Cooking Time: 10 minutes
Total Time: 40 minutes

Source
Source: Get Inspired Everyday

LAMB WITH OLIVE TAPENADE RICE

1/2 cup Kalamata olives, pitted
1 Tbs chopped fresh Oregano
1 Tbs Olive oil
3 cups Butternut squash, cubes
1 lb Ground lamb
1/2 tsp Cinnamon
1/2 tsp Sea salt

Procedure

1. Place olives, oregano, and olive oil in a food processor/blender and pulse until finely chopped. Set aside.
2. Now place butternut squash in the blender/processor (no need to wash it – yay!) and pulse until finely chopped. Set aside.
3. Heat a large skillet over medium-high heat. Add the ground lamb. Do not disturb for 4 minutes until the lamb is browned on one side. Now use a wooden spoon to break the meat into bite-sized chunks (size of mini meatballs). Flip each chunk and brown the other side for 2 minutes.
4. Add in the riced olives, butternut, cinnamon, and sea salt. Stir well, cover with a lid, and reduce heat to low. Cook for 5-6 more minutes. Serve warm.

Servings: 4

Preparation Time: 10 minutes
Cooking Time: 14 minutes

Source
Source: The Healing Kitchen cook book

LEMON & ASPARAGUS CHICKEN SKILLET

2 Tbs avocado oil

1 tsp sea salt, divided

1/2 tsp pepper, divided

1 lb chicken breast, cubed

1 bunch asparagus

3 cloves garlic, minced

1/3 cup chicken broth

Juice of one lemon

1 Tbs coconut aminos

1 tsp arrowroot starch

2 Tbs green onion, chopped

Procedure

1. Using a large skillet, heat the avocado oil on medium heat.
2. Add the chicken to the skillet and lightly season with salt and pepper. Cook until the chicken reaches an internal temperature of 165 F. Set aside.
3. Prepare the asparagus by chopping off the thick white base, and then slice in half again.
4. Add more oil to the pan if needed and saute the asparagus with more salt and pepper for about 5-7 minutes or until softened and lightly crisp. Set aside.
5. Reduce the heat slightly and add the minced garlic to the pan. Cook until fragrant.
6. Add the broth, lemon juice, coconut aminos, and arrowroot starch to the pan and stir for about 2-3 minutes or until the sauce lightly thickens.
7. Add the chicken and asparagus back to the pan and cook for another 2 minutes to reheat. 8 Serve topped with green onion and season further to taste.

Servings: 3

Preparation Time: 10 minutes

Cooking Time: 25 minutes

Total Time: 35 minutes

Source

Author: MICHELLE

Source: Unbound Wellness

MEDITERRANEAN CHICKEN WITH EGGPLANT

3 small eggplants, peeled and cut lengthwise into 1/2 inch thick slices
3 Tbs olive oil
6 skinless, boneless chicken breast halves - diced
1 onion, diced
2 Tbs tomato paste
½ cup water
2 tsp dried oregano
Salt and pepper to taste

Procedure

1. Place eggplant strips in a big pot of lightly salted water and soak for 30 minutes (this will improve the taste; they will leave a brown color in the pot).
2. Remove eggplant from pot and brush lightly with olive oil. Saute or grill until lightly browned and place in a 9x13 inch baking dish. Set aside.
3. Saute diced chicken and onion in a large skillet over medium heat. Stir in tomato paste and water, cover skillet, reduce heat to low and simmer for 10 minutes.
4. Preheat oven to 400 degrees F
5. Pour chicken/tomato mixture over eggplant. Season with oregano, salt and pepper and cover with aluminum foil. Bake in the pre heated oven for 20 minutes.

Servings: 6

Preparation Time: 50 minutes
Cooking Time: 30 minutes
Total Time: 1 hour and 20 minutes

Source
Source: Mediterranean Chicken with Eggplant
Web Page: All recipes

PALEO CHICKEN AND BROCCOLI

3 Tbs toasted sesame oil
7 cups broccoli cut into bite size pieces
2 Tbs grated ginger
1 tsp salt
1 tsp garlic powder
1 tsp red pepper flakes or to taste
2/3 cup coconut aminos
2 lbs chicken cut into bite-size pieces

Procedure

1. Place oil in a large skillet and add broccoli, ginger, salt, garlic powder, red pepper flakes and coconut aminos.
2. Cook over medium/high heat for 5 minutes until broccoli starts to soften.
3. Add the chicken and turn the heat to high.
4. Cook until chicken is fully cooked, stirring regularly, about 5 minutes.
5. If desired, add tapioca starch and stir well until sauce is thickened.
6. Serve over zucchini noodles or cauliflower rice.

Servings: 6

Cooking Time: 12 minutes

Source
Author: Real food with Jessica

PALEO CHICKEN PAD THAI

Not a detox friendly recipe, feel free to omit egg to make compliant.

FOR THE PAD THAI:
1 lb chicken breast or tenders*
Salt and pepper to taste

FOR THE SAUCE:
2 butternut squash bulbs
2 Tbs avocado or olive oil
1 red bell pepper chopped and de-seeded
2 carrots chopped or julienned
2 eggs
1/2 cup chopped red cabbage
1/4 cup chopped green onion
1/2 cup chopped almonds or cashews

1/4 chopped fresh cilantro optional
1/2 cup almond butter
1/3 cup cashew milk or your favorite dairy-free milk
3 Tbs rice syrup
1 Tbs toasted sesame oil
2 Tbs coconut aminos
2 cloves garlic crushed
1 tsp minced ginger
Juice of 1/2 lime

Procedure

1. Begin by heating your oven to 375 degrees. Line a baking sheet with foil and set aside.
2. Salt and pepper your chicken breasts (make sure they are roughly around the same size for even cooking). Place on the baking sheet.
3. Now prepare your butternut squash. Remove the bulbous end of the squash (you can't spiralize this end because of the seeds). Now peel the skin off the narrow end that you are going to spiralize. It's easier to cut this part in half. Spiralize the sized/shape noodles you like. (note that thicker noodles require at least 20-25 minutes, thinner noodles might be done faster). Once noodles are made, drizzle with a Tbsp of oil, add to the sheet pan. Salt and pepper both the chicken and the noodles. Place in the oven and bake for 20-25 minutes, or until chicken is cooked all the way.
4. Meanwhile make the sauce: in a blender or food processor, pulse together almond butter, rice syrup, sesame oil, coconut aminos,

garlic, lime, and ginger. While motor is running, pour in cashew milk. Continue to pulse until sauce is creamy and well combined.

5. Heat up skillet to medium heat. Spray with non-stick or use avocado oil. Saute carrots and bell pepper for 2-3 minutes. Whisk together eggs, and add them to the pan. Continue to cook another 2-3 minutes or until eggs are scrambled. Set aside.

6. Remove chicken and butternut squash noodles from the oven. Cut chicken into small pieces. Toss chicken and noodles into a large bowl. Now add in eggs and carrot/pepper mixture. Add in cabbage, cilantro, and cashews or almonds. Continue to toss and pour the sauce on top of the mixture (you may not want to use the entire sauce). Mix around until well combined.

7. Season with salt and pepper to taste. Serve!

Servings: 4

Preparation Time: 10 minutes
Cooking Time: 25 minutes
Total Time: 35 minutes

Source
Author: Amy
Source: wholesomelicious

Author Notes
*Chicken breast tenders are preferred since they will cook evenly. If you have just chicken breast, cut them into even strips.

PALEO SLOW COOKER INDIAN BUTTER CHICKEN

1 1/2 lb chicken breast, cubed
1 1/2 cup tomato sauce
1/2 cup chicken broth
2 Tbs ghee, melted (sub melted coconut oil)
1 1/2 tsp turmeric powder
3/4 tsp sea salt
1/4 tsp black pepper
1 tsp ground cumin
1 tsp chili powder
2 tsp garam masala
1 garlic clove, minced
2 tsp fresh ginger, grated
1/2 cup coconut cream Juice of one lime
2 Tbs fresh cilantro

Procedure

1. Add the chicken to the slow cooker. Add the tomato sauce, chicken broth, ghee and seasonings (reserving the cilantro) and stir well to thoroughly coat the chicken.
2. Set the lid on the slow cooker and cook on high for 1 1/2-2 hours or low for 4-6 hours, ensuring that the chicken has reached an internal temperature of 165 F.
3. Stir in the coconut cream and lime juice. Stir until melted and the sauce is creamy.
4. Serve topped with fresh cilantro with a side of rice or cauliflower rice.

Servings: 4

Preparation Time: 10 minutes
Cooking Time: 4 hours
Total Time: 4 hours and 10 minutes

Source
Author: MICHELLE
Source: Unbound wellness

Author Notes
This slow cooker Indian butter chicken is an easy and flavorful recipe that can be made into a speedy freezer meal!

To adapt for the freezer, add all of the ingredients (reserving ghee, coconut cream and cilantro to serve) to a freezer safe bag and freeze for 2-3 months. Allow to defrost fully and cook as directed. To adapt for the instant pot, use the poultry setting and ensure the chicken is fully cooked.

RANCH ROASTED CAULIFLOWER

1 Tbs dried parsley
1 Tbs garlic powder
1 Tbs onion powder
1 tsp dried dill
2 tsp dried chives
1 tsp salt
1/4 tsp black pepper
2 medium heads cauliflower, chopped into florets (about 6 cups)
3 Tbs avocado oil
1 Tbs fresh parsley, chopped (to serve)

Procedure

1. Preheat the oven to 400 F and line a baking sheet with parchment paper.
2. Prepare the ranch blend with parsley, garlic, onion powder, dill, chives, salt and pepper. Set aside
3. Add the cauliflower to the baking sheet and top with the avocado oil and ranch blend. Toss to combine.
4. Transfer to the oven and bake for 35-40 minutes (or until crisped to your liking), rotating halfway through.
5. Serve topped with fresh parsley.

Source
Author: MICHELLE
Source: Unbound Wellness

SALMON BURGERS WITH AVOCADO AIOLI

To make detox diet friendly substitution for 2 eggs: 2 tablespoons chia seed 5 teaspoons water, mix and let rest

2 6 ounce cans canned salmon

2 eggs, lightly beaten * see note for egg substitute

1/2 tsp garlic powder (or 2 fresh cloves, crushed)

2 Tbs fresh herbs – finely chopped (dill, parsley, basil, and/or cilantro)

2 Tbs lemon juice

1/2 tsp lemon zest

1/4 cup almond flour

Salt and pepper to taste

1 Tbs ghee or avocado oil for cooking

FOR AVOCADO AIOLI

1 ripe avocado

1/4 cup sugar free Mayonnaise

2 Tbs fresh cilantro, roughly chopped

2 Tbs lime juice

1/2 tsp garlic powder

Salt to taste

Butter lettuce, arugula for base of meal

Procedure

1. In a bowl, combine salmon, eggs, garlic powder, fresh herbs, lemon juice, lemon zest, almond flour, salt, and pepper until well incorporated.
2. Form 4 patties and set aside.
3. Heat large skillet over medium-high heat and add cooking fat. Once pan is nice and hot, gently add salmon burgers and turn heat down to medium. Cook for 4-5 minutes, until golden on bottom. Flip and cook another 4- 5 minutes until cooked all the way through and golden.
4. While burgers cook, prepare avocado aioli by processing all aioli ingredients in a food processor or blender until creamy smooth.
5. Serve salmon burgers over crisp butter lettuce and arugula. Top with avocado aioli. Maybe add some pickled red onions. Enjoy!

Source
Author: Savory Lotus

SHEET PAN LEMON CHICKEN AND ASPARAGUS

4 bone-in chicken thighs (about 1.5 lbs)
1 large white sweet potato, finely cubed (sub orange sweet potatoes)
3 Tbs avocado oil, divided
1– 1 1/2 tsp sea salt, divided

1/2 tsp black pepper
1 bunch asparagus, trimmed
2 cloves garlic, minced
1 large lemon, juiced
3–4 slices of fresh lemon
2 Tbs parsley, chopped

Procedure

1. Preheat the oven to 400 F and line a large baking sheet with parchment paper.
2. Pat the chicken thighs dry.
3. Add the sweet potato to one half of the baking sheet, and the chicken to the other. Top with 2 tbsp of avocado oil, salt and pepper. Roast in the oven for 25-30 minutes, turning the sweet potato halfway through to evenly bake.
4. Remove from the oven and use a spatula to make room for the asparagus. Add the asparagus to the pan and top with more avocado oil, salt and pepper. Add the garlic, lemon juice, and lemon slices to the rest of the sheet pan.
5. Bake in the oven for 10-15 more minutes or until the vegetables are cooked to your liking and the chicken reads an internal temperature of 165 F.
6. Serve topped with fresh parsley and more seasoning to taste.

Servings: 4

Preparation Time: 10 minutes
Cooking Time: 45 minutes
Total Time: 55 minutes

Source
Author: MICHELLE
Source: Unbound Wellness

SHEET PAN LEMON-HERB LAMB & VEGGIES

FOR MEATBALLS:

1 lb ground lamb   *
1 tsp minced fresh thyme 1 tsp sea salt   *
3 minced garlic cloves Zest of 1 lemon   *

FOR VEGGIES:

1 head cauliflower, chopped into   2 Tbs olive oil
florets   2 tsp minced fresh thyme
1 head bok choy, chopped, washed,   1 tsp sea salt
and dried   Juice of 1 lemon
1 eggplant largely diced

Procedure

1. Preheat oven to 400 degrees F. Line a large baking sheet with parchment paper. Set aside.
2. By hand in a medium bowl, mix all the meatball ingredients together thoroughly. Form into 12 meatballs. Set aside.
3. Using a wooden spoon in a large bowl, mix all the veggie ingredients together until all the veggies are well coated with oil and seasonings. Spread veggie mixture out evenly over the baking sheet.
4. Place meatballs evenly spaced among the veggies.
5. Bake for 30 minutes. Serve warm.

Servings: 4

Preparation Time: 15 minutes
Cooking Time: 30 minutes
Total Time: 45 minutes

Source
Author: Angie Alt
Source: Modified from AutoImmune Wellness

SHEET PAN TURKEY DINNER

12 oz green beans (cleaned and trimmed)
2 Tbs olive oil
1 shallot (peeled, halved and cut into thin slices)
salt and pepper
1 lb sweet potatoes (peeled and cut into ½-inch cubes)

½ tsp salt
⅛ tsp cinnamon
24 oz turkey tenderloin (cut into 4 equal pieces with silver skin trimmed off)
2 cloves garlic (minced)
½ tsp dried rosemary
¼ tsp dried sage

Procedure

1. Preheat the oven to 375° F. Arrange green beans evenly on the sheet pan. Drizzle with 1 tablespoon of olive oil, sprinkle ½ teaspoon of salt, ¼ teaspoon of pepper, 1 clove of minced garlic and the shallots. Gently toss to coat.
2. In a medium mixing bowl, toss together the sweet potatoes, 1 tablespoon olive oil, ½ teaspoon salt and the cinnamon. Arrange sweet potatoes evenly with the green beans on the sheet pan.
3. In the same bowl, add turkey ½ teaspoon salt, ¼ teaspoon pepper, rosemary, sage and remaining garlic. Toss the turkey in the bowl until the seasoning is evenly coating the turkey. Arrange the four pieces into the veggies evenly down the pan.
4. Bake in the oven for 25 minutes or until the turkey juices run clear and an instant read thermometer reads 165° F when placed in the center.
5. Allow to cool for 5 minutes and serve warm or refrigerate for up to 5 days, freeze for up to 60 days.

Servings: 4

Preparation Time: 10 minutes
Cooking Time: 25 minutes
Total Time: 35 minutes

SHREDDED PUMPKIN CHICKEN

1 Tbs fat of choice (duck fat or avocado oil are great)
1 shallot, sliced
5 cloves of garlic, pressed or grated
4 chicken breasts, bones and skin removed
1 tsp salt

1/2 tsp garlic powder
1 15 oz can pumpkin puree
1 cup bone broth (homemade or store bought)
1 tsp dried rosemary
1/2 tsp dried thyme

Procedure

1. In the bottom of your pressure cooker, heat fat over medium heat. Add shallot and cook to soften some, stirring occasionally – about 4 minutes. Add the garlic and stir.
2. Season the chicken breasts liberally with salt and garlic powder. Add to the pressure cooker.
3. Add pureed pumpkin, bone broth, and remaining seasonings. Stir to combine.
4. Place your lid on the pressure cooker, lock, and bring to high pressure. Continue cooking while maintaining high pressure for 25 minutes. Let the pressure naturally release.
5. Carefully remove the lid once the pressure release valve has lowered. Check to be sure the chicken is cooked through (thicker breasts may need longer) and shred the chicken with the pumpkin sauce. 6 Serve immediately with your favorite seasonal side dishes.

Servings: 4

Preparation Time: 10 minutes
Cooking Time: 25 minutes
Total Time: 35 minutes

Source
Author: Erin
Source: Real food and Love

Author Notes

Slow cooker method:

Place all ingredients in the crock of your slow cooker.

Toss to combine and cook on low for 4 hours.

Carefully remove chicken and shred with the pumpkin sauce.

Serve immediately with your favorite seasonal side dishes.

SLOW COOKER MONGOLIAN BEEF

1 1/2 lb flank steak, sliced thin against the grain
1 tsp sea salt
1/4 tsp black pepper
1 Tbs arrowroot starch
1/2 cup carrots, shredded
2 tsp rice syrup

1/2 cup coconut aminos
1/2 cup beef broth (sub water)
2 tsp lime Juice
3 cloves garlic, minced
1 Tbs ginger, grated
3-4 green onions, sliced into 1" pieces

Procedure

1. Season the beef with salt and pepper and toss in arrowroot starch to thoroughly coat. Add to the bottom of the slow cooker along with the carrots.
2. Combine the coconut aminos, rice syrup, broth, lime juicer, and seasonings (reserving the green onion) and mix well.
3. Pour the mixture into the slow cooker and stir well to coat.
4. Place the lid on the slow cooker and cook on high for 2-3 hours or low for 4-5 hours.
5. Stir in the green onion and allow to soften.
6. Serve with cauliflower rice or steamed broccoli.

Servings: 6

Preparation Time: 10 minutes
Cooking Time: 2 hours

Source
Author: MICHELLE
Source: Unbound Wellness

SLOW COOKER POT ROAST

2 Tbs avocado oil
3 lb boneless beef chuck roast boneless
1 tsp salt, divided
1/2 tsp black pepper
4 cloves garlic, minced
1/2 yellow onion, diced
2 cups carrots, peeled and chopped
2 cups parsnip, peeled and chopped

1 Tbs rosemary leaves, chopped
2 tsp fresh thyme leaves
3 bay leaves
1 3/4 cups beef broth
2 Tbs coconut aminos
1 Tbs arrowroot starch
2 Tbs parsley, chopped

Procedure

1. Using a large pan, heat the avocado oil over medium heat. Add the roast, season with salt and pepper, and sear for 2-3 minutes on each side or until lightly browned. Remove from the pan and place on the bottom of the slow cooker.

2. Add the onion and garlic to the pan and saute for 3-4 minutes or until slightly translucent. Remove from the pan and add to the slow cooker.

3. Add the parsnip, carrots, rosemary, thyme, bay leaves, broth & coconut aminos to the slow cooker. Place the lid on the slow cooker and cook on low for 7 hours.

4. Once finished, spoon out about 1 cup of liquid into a bowl. Whisk in the arrowroot starch until fully combined. Add back to the slow cooker and allow to cook for another hour.

5. Turn off the slow cooker and remove the bay leaves.

6. Serve the roast shredded along with the vegetables and gravy

Servings: 6

Cooking Time: 8 hours
Total Time: 8 hours and 15 minutes

Source
Author: MICHELLE
Source: Unbound Wellness

Author Notes
To adapt for the instant pot, cook on high pressure for 60 minutes, and add arrowroot starch at the end after you remove the lid to thicken the broth.

SLOW-COOKER PALEO MEATBALLS FOR MEATBALLS

FOR SAUCE

1 1/2 lb ground beef

1/4 cup freshly chopped parsley, plus more for garnish

2 1/2 tsp water

1 Tbsp chia seed

2 garlic cloves, minced

1 tsp kosher salt

1/2 tsp crushed red pepper flakes

1 (28-oz.) can crushed tomatoes

1 (6-oz.) can tomato paste

1/4 yellow onion, finely chopped

2 tsp dried oregano

1 garlic clove, minced

Kosher salt

Freshly ground black pepper

Procedure

1. Mix together 1 Tbsp Chia seeds and 2 1/2 tsp water, let rest to thicken.
2. Make meatballs: In a large bowl, mix together beef, parsley, chia seed egg substitute, garlic, salt, and red pepper flakes until combined. Form mixture into 24 meatballs and place in slow cooker.
3. Make sauce: In another large bowl, stir together crushed tomatoes, tomato paste, onion, oregano, and garlic and season with salt and pepper. Pour over meatballs.
4. Cook, covered, on low until meatballs are cooked through, 5 to 5 1/2 hours.
5. Garnish with parsley before serving.

Yield: 24

Preparation Time: 15 minutes
Cooking Time: 5 hours and 45 minutes
Total Time: 5 hours and 45 minutes

Source
Author: Delish

TURKEY PESTO MEATBALLS

PESTO INGREDIENTS

1 cup arugula

1 cup fresh basil

1/2 cup olive oil

3 Tbs fresh lemon juice

1 clove of garlic, peeled and minced

1/2 tsp sea salt

*

*

FOR THE MEATBALLS

2 Tbs olive oil, divided

1/4 white onion, diced

3 cloves garlic, minced

1 lb ground turkey

2 Tbs coconut flour

2 Tbs fresh basil, chopped

1/2 tsp sea salt

1/4 tsp black pepper

Procedure

1. For the pesto
2. Using a high speed blender, blend all of the ingredients until smooth. Set aside in the fridge.
3. For the meatballs
4. Preheat the oven to 375 F and line a baking sheet with parchment paper. Set aside
5. Using a medium pan, heat 1 tbsp of olive oil over medium-low heat. Saute the onion for 3-4 minutes or until lightly translucent. Add the garlic and saute for another 2 minutes. Set aside and allow to cool slightly.
6. Add the ground turkey, basil, coconut flour, salt, pepper, along with the remainder of the olive oil and onion and garlic mixture in a bowl and mix well to combine.
7. Form the mixture into meatballs and place on the baking sheet.
8. Bake in the preheated oven for 30-35 minutes, flipping halfway through. The internal temperature should read 165 F.
9. Serve topped with pesto and a side of vegetables.

Servings: 4

Source
Author: MICHELLE
Source: Unbound Wellness

TURKEY PUMPKIN MEATBALLS WITH CREAMY HARVEST TOMATO SAUCE

Not a detox friendly recipe, to make compliant substitute for egg- mix 1 tablespoon chia seed and 2 1/2 teaspoons water, let rest.

MEATBALLS:
1.25 lbs ground turkey
1/2 cup organic pumpkin puree
1/4 cup blanched almond flour
3/4 tsp salt
1/8 tsp black pepper

1 egg *egg substitute see above
1 Tbs fresh thyme minced
1 Tbs fresh sage minced
1 Tbs fresh rosemary minced

SAUCE:
2 Tbs organic coconut oil or ghee
15 oz can tomato sauce
1 1/4 cups organic pumpkin puree or remaining amount from a 15 oz can
1/2 cup full fat coconut milk see note below**
1/2 cup chicken bone broth or homemade bone broth

1 small Onion chopped
3 cloves Garlic minced
2 tsp Italian seasoning
1 tsp pumpkin pie spice optional
1/2 tsp dried sage
1/2 tsp dried crushed rosemary
Salt and black pepper to taste
Crushed red pepper optional, for spice
Chopped parsley for garnish

Procedure

1. To make meatballs:
2. Preheat your oven to 425 degrees F and line a large baking sheet with parchment paper.
3. Mix all meatball ingredients in a large bowl with your hands until well combined. Form mixture into 18 balls see note below*
4. Bake meatballs on baking sheet at 425 for 15-18 minutes or until no longer pink on the inside, turning once midway.
5. To Make Sauce:
6. Meanwhile, melt the coconut oil or ghee in a large saucepan or stock pot over medium heat. Add the onions and cook until translucent

and fragrant, then add the garlic and continue to cook for 2 minutes or until soft and fragrant.

7. Lower the heat, then add the tomato sauce, pumpkin, broth, coconut milk, Italian seasoning, pumpkin pie spice, dried sage, dried rosemary and stir to combine well. Season with salt, black pepper or crushed red pepper, if desired. Stir to combine flavors, then cover and allow to simmer for 5 minutes prior to adding the meatballs.

8. Add the meatballs and continue to simmer on low heat for about 5 minutes prior to serving.

9. Serve over your favorite veggie noodles (I love sweet potato noodles with these!)

Servings: 6

Preparation Time: 15 minutes
Cooking Time: 25 minutes
Total Time: 40 minutes

Source
Author: Michele Rosen

Author Notes
*If your mixture is sticky, wet your hands a bit before rolling into balls, as needed. **Blend your coconut milk to a smooth consistency before adding. If you prefer a slightly thinner sauce, use 1/4 cup coconut milk and 3/4 cup broth instead of 1/2 and 1/2.

ZUCCHINI NOODLES WITH SCALLOPS & BACON

1 lb petite bay scallops, cleaned & rinsed
6 slices uncured bacon sugar free
8 medium zucchini
2 tsp garlic powder
6 green onions, sliced with green tops reserved for garnish
Squeeze fresh lemon juice
Sea salt & fresh black pepper to taste

Procedure

1. Lay the cleaned scallops on a clean dish towel or paper towel to dry. Fold the clean towel over the scallops or lay an extra sheet of paper towel on top. Press gently to absorb excess moisture; set aside, still covered.
2. In a large flat bottomed pan, cook the bacon until crisp.
3. While the bacon is cooking, use a vegetable spiralizer or julienne peeler to make your zucchini noodles. Save the noodles for later.
4. When the bacon is cooked, remove from the pan and set it aside.
5. Pour off most of the excess bacon fat and save for later, leaving behind just enough to coat the pan lightly. Save the pan to cook the scallops later.
6. In a large, high sided pan, add about 2 tsp of the reserved bacon fat. Bring to medium high heat and add the zucchini noodles and garlic powder. Season to taste with salt and pepper.
7. Saute the zucchini noodles until just softened, about 3 – 5 minutes. While the noodles are cooking, chop the cooked reserved bacon into pieces.
8. Remove the noodles from the heat and toss them with 2/3 of the bacon, the white parts of the chopped green onions and a squeeze of lemon juice. Set to one side.
9. Return the flat bottomed pan to the stove and bring to medium high heat. Add the dried scallops to the pan; they should sizzle straight away, but the bacon fat should not be so hot it is smoking.

10. Sear the scallops until golden brown on the bottom, about 2 minutes. Toss or flip the scallops and sear the other side for 1 – 2 minutes, until golden.
11. Remove the scallops from the heat and toss them in with the noodles.
12. Divide the noodles between plates and garnish with the remaining bacon pieces and green onions.

Cooking Time: 30 minutes
Total Time: 30 minutes

Source
Author: Meatified

DR. BUMP'S LUNCH RECIPES

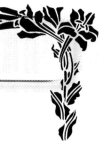

CAULIFLOWER TORTILLAS

¾ a head of cauliflower riced or 2 cups riced and packed

2 eggs

Salt and pepper to taste

Procedure

1. Preheat oven to 375 degrees and line a baking tray with parchment paper.
2. For these I actually rice my cauliflower slightly more fine that cauliflower rice. Toss ¾ a head of cauliflower cut up and most of the stem removed and pulse until you get a texture slightly finer than rice. (Once it's riced measure it to make sure you have 2 cups packed.)
3. Place riced cauliflower in bowl and microwave for 2 minutes and stir, then another two minutes and stir again then place in a dish towel and squeeze excess water out as hard as you can. (You're going to want to get out as much water as you can and be careful not to burn yourself because it's going to be very hot.)
4. Place drained cauliflower back in bowl and add two eggs, salt and pepper and mix until well combined.
5. As a note it will be a little bit runny but shouldn't be pure liquid either. Spread mixture onto a baking sheet into 6 small fairly flat circles.
6. Place in the oven for 10 minutes then pull out of the oven and carefully peel them off the parchment and flip them and place back in the oven for 5-7 more minutes.
7. Once they're done place them on a wire rack to cool slightly.
8. Heat a medium sized pan over medium heat and place the tortillas into the pan pressing down slightly and brown them to your liking. (Don't skip this step because it gives them slightly crispy on the edges and gives them a wonderfully nutty taste)

Servings: 6

Preparation Time: 10 minutes
Cooking Time: 17 minutes
Total Time: 27 minutes

Source
Author: Joshua
Source: Slim palate

CREATE YOUR OWN SALAD

Start with your choice of salad Fixings

2 cups Leafy greens: spinach, romaine, Spring greens, radicchio, arugula, iceberg, kale

1-2 cups Add some Vegetables: tomatoes, peppers, celery, onion, cucumber, artichoke, scallion, radish etc. 2-4 ounces

Add some protein: Chicken, turkey, beef, ham, shrimp, tuna, crab meat, crispy bacon, hard cooked egg

Procedure

1. Try these variations
2. CHEF STYLE
3. Ounce lean cooked roast beef, Turkey breast or chicken breast
4. One hard boiled egg
5. NICOISE STYLE
6. Quarter cup water packed tuna
7. One hard cooked egg
8. Six large olives
9. Half a cup green beans

EGG ROLL IN A BOWL

2 Tbs olive oil divided
1 lb ground turkey or beef 93/7
1 ½ cup sweet onion finely diced
1 cup carrots shredded
½ tsp ginger minced
3 cloves garlic crushed
¼ cup chicken broth
5 cups cabbage cut into ¼-inch shreds

2 Tbs coconut aminos
2 tsp lime juice
½ tsp salt to taste
¼ tsp pepper to taste
1 tsp toasted sesame oil
Toasted sesame seeds optional
Green onions optional

Procedure

1. In a large saute pan over medium heat drizzle 1 tablespoon olive oil and add ground turkey. Cook for 5-6 minutes, or until turkey is almost cooked through.
2. Push turkey to the side of the pan and add onion and other tablespoon of oil. Saute for 3-4 minutes.
3. Add shredded carrots, garlic, and ginger and saute for 2 minutes. Stir the vegetables and turkey together.
4. Pour chicken broth in the pan and scrape the bottom of it to deglaze it.
5. Add cabbage, coconut aminos, lime juice, salt, and pepper. Stir well and cover with a lid. Reduce heat to medium-low and cook for 12-15 minutes, or until cabbage is to your desired tenderness.
6. Just before serving add toasted sesame oil and top with green onions and toasted sesame seeds. Serve over cauliflower rice, or eat it in a bowl by itself. Enjoy!

Servings: 4

Preparation Time: 10 minutes
Cooking Time: 20 minutes
Total Time: 30 minutes

Source
Author: Evolving Table

GRAIN FREE CAULIFLOWER TABBOULEH SALAD

1/4 cup olive oil

3 Tbs lemon juice

1 tsp sea salt

1/4 tsp black pepper

1 clove garlic, minced

2 1/2 cups cauliflower, riced

1/4 cup red onion, diced

1/4 cup tomato, diced

1/4 cup cucumber, diced

2 Tbs fresh dill, chopped

3 Tbs fresh mint, chopped

1/3 cup parsley, chopped

Procedure

1. Using a small bowl, whisk the olive oil, lemon juice, salt, pepper, and garlic together. Set aside.
2. Add the remainder of the ingredients to a large bowl and toss to combine. Add the oil and lemon mixture and stir to combine.
3. Season further to taste and serve fresh.

Source
Author: MICHELLE
Source: Unbound Wellness

GRILLED CHICKEN & ROMAINE WITH CREAMY AVOCADO CAESAR DRESSING

Ingredients

2 Pkgs organic Boneless Skinless   *
Chicken Breasts (total of 4 pieces)   *
Himalayan Salt   *
Black Pepper   *
2 Romaine Lettuce Hearts   *
1 or 2 Lemons for grilling and   *
seasoning, cut in half or quarters
(optional)

MARINADE:

4 Tbs Extra Virgin Olive Oil   1 Lemon, juiced
2 cloves Garlic, chopped or minced   2 Tbs Parsley, chopped (optional)

CREAMY AVOCADO CAESAR DRESSING:

2 Avocados, peeled and pitted   2 Lemons, juiced
6 cloves Garlic, minced   1/2 tsp Anchovy Paste (optional
1/2 cup Extra Virgin Olive Oil   but recommended)
1/2 tsp Himalayan Salt, or to taste

Procedure

1. Mix all marinade ingredients together in a shallow glass dish. Arrange chicken in a single layer and allow to marinade for a total of 30 minutes (15 minutes in the refrigerator and 15 minutes at room temperature) – While your chicken is marinating, prepare the dressing.

2. Add all dressing ingredients to a deep bowl or large liquid measuring cup and blend well using a stick/immersion blender. If your dressing is too thick, blend in ½ tsp of water (or additional lemon juice – test for flavor before you decide) at a time until you reach your desired consistency.

3. Refrigerate and allow the flavors to meld.

4. Trim and discard the root end of the romaine lettuce, removing only as much as necessary so the head remains intact. Cut the romaine in half lengthwise and rinse under cold running water (do not soak). Wrap the romaine in paper towels or a clean kitchen towel to remove excess water.

5. Bring chicken to room temperature approximately 15 minutes before grilling, this will help ensure your meat cooks more evenly.

6. Preheat indoor or outdoor grill to high heat.

7. Remove chicken breasts from marinade and place on pre-heated grill. Season with salt and pepper. Place halved or quartered lemons cut side down on grill.

8. Allow chicken breasts to cook over high heat until they release easily from grill, about 5 minutes. Turn chicken breasts over, season again with salt and pepper and allow to cook on second side until chicken releases easily from grill.

9. Continue grilling lemon cut side down as chicken cooks. Cook lemon until slightly softened and grill marks have formed, about 5 minutes. Remove lemons from the grill and let stand.

10. Continuing grilling chicken, turning and moving until cooked through and an internal temperature of 165F has been reached. Remove chicken from grill and allow to rest, tented with foil, for a few minutes before slicing.

11. While the chicken is resting, place the washed and dried romaine hearts cut side down on the grill, cook until grill marks form, about 3 minutes. Gently turn the lettuce using tongs, and grill for an additional 2 minutes. Remove from grill.

12. Plate your grilled romaine, top with chicken slices breast, a drizzle of Avocado Caesar Dressing and the grilled lemon on the side. Add a squeeze of grilled lemon to your salad and enjoy!

Servings: 4

Preparation Time: 15 minutes
Cooking Time: 15 minutes
Total Time: 45 minutes

GROUND BEEF TACO SALAD

FOR THE TACO GROUND BEEF

1 Tbs olive oil

1.5 lbs lean ground beef — preferably grass-fed, organic

1 cup white onion — diced

½ cup red bell pepper

3 cloves garlic — minced

1 tsp paprika

1 Tbs onion powder

1 tsp coriander powder

1 tsp chili powder

1 tsp cumin powder

1 Tbs dried oregano

1/2 tsp cayenne pepper — optional

Salt and ground black pepper to taste

1 cup chicken broth

FOR THE SALSA

2 medium tomatoes — diced

¼ cup red onion — diced

1 green bell pepper — diced

1 tsp jalapeno — chopped (remove seeds for less heat)

Fresh cilantro — chopped (optional)

1 Tbs fresh lime juice

1 small garlic clove — minced

Salt and pepper to taste

FOR THE SALAD

4-6 cups romaine lettuce — chopped

half avocado — sliced

lime wedges – for garnish

salt and pepper to taste

cilantro for garnish

Procedure

1. FOR THE TACO GROUND BEEF
2. In a large pot or Dutch oven, heat olive oil over high heat. Add the ground beef and cook it until it gets completely brown. Set it aside.
3. Reduce the heat to medium-low, add onion and bell pepper. Cook until onions are soft and translucent, about 5 to 8 minutes.
4. Add garlic and sauté for 30 seconds. Add all the spices (paprika, onion powder, coriander powder, chili powder, cumin powder, dried oregano, cayenne pepper, salt and black pepper).
5. Stir everything together and bring cooked ground beef to the pot. Give a stir and add chicken stock.

6. Bring the ground beef mixture to a boil and then, lower the heat to low, cover with a lid and cook 30-60 min (the longer, the better), stirring occasionally to avoid burning.
7. FOR THE SALSA
8. Combine all the ingredients in a bowl. Cover tightly and refrigerate for up to 5 days.
9. FOR THE SALAD
10. In a large salad bowl, add lettuces, sliced avocado, salsa and 1/4 of the cooked ground beef.
11. Squeeze some lime on top of the salad and season it with salt and pepper if necessary.
12. Garnish with fresh cilantro. Enjoy!

Servings: 4

Preparation Time: 10 minutes
Cooking Time: 15 minutes
Total Time: 20 minutes

Source
Source: Primavera Kitchen

QUICK CAULIFLOWER FRIED "RICE"

This dish can be be made meatless.

1 pound ground pork
1 Onion chopped
4 celery stalks chopped
1 red pepper diced
1/2 cauliflower head
1/4 cabbage
4 large carrots
2 large broccoli - stems & flowers separated
1/2 cup snow peas. sliced

3 cloves garlic — minced
2 Tbsp ginger grated
2-3 Tbsp avocado oil
1/2 tsp sesame oil
1/4 cup coconut amonos
2 tbsp almond butter
1-2 Tbsp water
1/4 cup chopped cashews for garnish
1/4 cup scallions, sliced thin crosswise

Procedure

1. Brown ground pork in 1 Tablespoon avocado oil in large frying pan
2. Meanwhile using food processor large shred blade, shred the cauliflower flowers, cabbage, carrot & broccoli stems only
3. Once pork is browned, remove from pan & put aside
4. Add remaining avocado oil to pan and saute onion, celery and red pepper stirring occasionally, until softened but not browned
5. Add garlic and ginger and stir for 30 seconds
6. Add cauliflower rice, broccoli stems & cabbage to pan and cook stirring until vegetables are cooked.
7. Meanwhile add the almond butter, water, coconut aminos and sesame oil in small bowl and whisk
8. During the last 5 minutes of cooking add the cooked pork, mini broccoli flowers & sliced snow peas
9. Pour the aminos almond butter mixture over pan and stir to combine cook 5 more minutes
10. Garnish with chopped cashews and scallions

Source
Author: Victoria

SALMON PATTIES WITH A CREAMY LEMON-DILL SAUCE

This recipe is not detox compliant

2 (6-ounce) cans of wild salmon
4 eggs
1 Tbs of mustard
1 cup of almond flour
4 cloves of garlic, minced

1 onion, finely diced
1/2 tsp pepper
1/2 tsp salt (optional)
1 tsp dill
2-4 TB of coconut oil/or butter/or lard

CREAMY LEMON-DILL SAUCE
1/2 cup of thick, full-fat coconut milk (I used the thick part off an unshaken can)
2 Tbs of lemon juice
1 tsp of dried dill
Few shakes of black pepper

Procedure

1. CREAMY DILL SAUCE
2. Whisk all the ingredients together. Pour over the Salmon Patties and enjoy!
3. Preheat a cast iron skillet over medium heat with your fat/oil of choice.
4. In a bowl, whisk your eggs, then add the onions, garlic, almond flour, salmon, pepper, salt, dill, and mustard.
5. Shape into 8 patties. Fry them on both sides; about 3-4 minutes per side.
6. Transfer to a plate. Put them in the oven for an additional 10 minutes (450 degrees F) while you make the cream sauce. This will make sure the middle is cooked through.

Source
Author: The Paleo Mama

SHEET PAN VEGGIES

4 Small Heads of Baby Bok Choy
3 carrots (diced, 1 cup)
4 hands full of brussel sprouts
2 Tbs avocado oil

pinch sea salt garlic powder to taste
onion powder to taste
ginger powder is desired black
pepper

Procedure

1. Instructions
2. Remove the bottom of the Bok Choy and then cut it in half and then in thin strips or after cutting the bottom off, continue to chop it from the bottom all the way through to the green tops.
3. Slice carrots into thin ribbons using a mandolin slicer or veggie peeler. You could spiralize them if you like.
4. Slice brussel sprouts thinly
5. Spread your veggies on a parchment lined baking sheet (parchment makes for easy clean-up).
6. Drizzle with Avocado Oil. I prefer avocado for its higher smoke point)
7. Sprinkle with a pinch of Himalayan Salt (go easy - it doesn't take much to over-salt veggies cooked like this)
8. Since I add so little of each of the garlic, onion and optional ginger powder (depending on what vegetables you're using or what you're serving it with you may not want to use ginger) and pepper, I don't include measurements - just a light sprinkle over the sheet of vegetables.
9. Use your hands to massage oil and spices through the veggies.
10. ROASTING - I typically cook this recipe at the same time as my main dish, and have found it works well at a variety of temps and durations. I look along with salmon for 20 mins at 400 degrees. If you've got something going at a higher temp and longer cooking time, just toss the pan in at about 15-20 mins before your cooking time is up.

Preparation Time: 5 minutes
Cooking Time: 20 minutes
Total Time: 25 minutes

Source
Source: AIPRecipeCollection.com

Author Notes
More Veggie Suggestions!
You could use onions, broccoli, cauliflower, zucchini, parsnips, sweet potatoes, kale or chard too. Use your imagination. Adjust veggies and quantities to your preference. Just be sure to slice your veg in reasonable sizes to allow them to cook properly.

THAI PORK LETTUCE WRAPS

1 lb finely diced pork
2 cups chicken stock
3/4 lb mung bean sprouts
Fresh lettuce leaves, cut into
approximately 3 x 3 inches
½ cup almond butter
1 Tbs fish sauce

1 Tbs lemon juice
4 Tbs of water
1 lime, quartered
1 Tbs olive oil
Sea salt and freshly ground black
pepper to taste;

Procedure

1. Bring the chicken stock to a boil in a pan placed over a medium-high heat and add the pork slices. Simmer and cook for about 5 minutes, until the pork is cooked.
2. Remove the pork pieces and set aside to cool. You won't need the chicken stock anymore, but you can store it in the refrigerator for later recipes.
3. In the same pan, cook the mung bean sprouts with the cooking fat for 3 to 4 minutes and then set aside.
4. In a bowl, combine the ingredients for the almond butter sauce: the almond butter, fish sauce, lemon juice & water. Season to taste with sea salt and black pepper.
5. Once the cooked ingredients have cooled down, place some pork, some mung bean sprouts and some almond butter sauce over each lettuce leaf and squeeze some fresh lime juice on top. Roll them into wraps and enjoy.

Servings: 4

Preparation Time: 10 minutes

Source
Author: Paleo Leap

THAI TURKEY BURGERS

1 lb ground turkey
½ cup shredded carrots
1 Tbs chopped cilantro
1 green onion, chopped

½ tsp salt
½ tsp garlic powder
½ tsp ground ginger
1 Tbs olive oil or avocado oil

ALMOND BUTTER SAUCE:
2 Tbs almond butter
1 Tbs coconut aminos

1 Tbs lime Juice

COLESLAW:
2 Tbs almond butter
2 Tbs lime Juice
2 Tbs coconut aminos
1 Tbs water
½ tsp garlic powder

1 tsp sesame oil
1/4 tsp ground ginger 10 oz bag of
coleslaw mix
1 Tbs chopped cilantro
1 head of cabbage

Procedure

1. In a medium sized bowl combine 2 tablespoons almond butter, 2 Tablespoons lime juice, 2 tablespoons coconut aminos, 1 tablespoon water, ½ teaspoon garlic powder, 1 teaspoon sesame oil and ¼ teaspoon ground ginger. Whisk to fully combine then add in coleslaw mix and cilantro and toss to coat.
2. In a bowl combine turkey, shredded carrots, 1 tablespoon cilantro, green onion, salt, garlic powder and ground ginger. Mix with your hands or a wooden spoon to fully combine.
3. Divide into 4 pieces and form the pieces into patties (about the size of your palm). Turn your grill or pan on medium high heat and once the pan is hot, add oil. Place patties on the pan and cook for about 4 minutes per side, until they reach an internal temperature of 165°F. Remove and set aside.
4. In a small bowl combine all of the almond butter sauce ingredients and set aside.
5. To make burger, peel off leaves of cabbage and top with a burger patty, some almond butter sauce and coleslaw!

Source
Author: KELSEY

TUNA SALAD

1 can or jar wild caught tuna
1 can non GMO artichoke hearts
chopped finely (or run through
food processor)

2 stalks celery chopped
1/4 whole onion (diced, 1 cup)
15 kalamata olives pitted and sliced
2-3 Tbsp sugar free Mayonnaise

Procedure

1 mix everything together and put on top of salad or in lettuce cups

Yield: 3 to 4 servings

Source
Author: Victoria

ZUCCHINI BOATS

3 Medium/Large Zucchini
Extra Virgin Olive Oil

Himalayan Salt
Black Pepper

FILLING

1 Tbs Extra Virgin Olive Oil
1 Small Onion, diced
2 cloves Garlic, minced
1 lb Lean Grass-Fed Ground Beef
Reserved Zucchini (from step 1), chopped

1 Medium Carrot, finely shredded
1 Tbs Dried Oregano
1 Tbs Dried Basil
1 Tbs Dried Parsley
1/2 tsp Himalayan Salt
1 tsp Garlic Powder
1 tsp Onion Powder

TOPPING

1/2 cup Green Onions, thinly sliced
2 Tbs Extra Virgin Olive Oil

Procedure

1. Wash zucchini and trim ends off. Slice in half length-wise and scoop out the insides to create a boat/cavity deep enough to allow space for your meat mixture. Reserve the zucchini you scoop out.
2. Place zucchini boats in a Pyrex baking dish or casserole dish and brush lightly with olive oil. Sprinkle with pinch of salt and black pepper.
3. Mix ground beef, chopped reserved zucchini, shredded carrot and the dry seasonings. Use your hands to ensure everything is well blended.
4. In a large skillet, heat 1 Tbsp olive oil and saute onion until translucent. Add minced garlic and saute until fragrant.
5. Preheat oven to 400 F.
6. Add ground beef mixture and saute until browned. If there is a lot of fat, you can drain it off, I didn't find the need.
7. Spoon filling mixture into zucchini boats and add the topping mixture. Sprinkle with extra dried parsley if you wish, and a pinch or two of black pepper.

8. Bake at 400 F for 25 minutes or until zucchini are tender but still al dente in texture. You can opt to broil for a few minutes to ensure the topping is browned and crispy.

9. Serve immediately.

Preparation Time: 10 minutes
Cooking Time: 25 minutes
Total Time: 35 minutes

Source
Source: AIPRecipeCollection.com

ZUCCHINI NOODLES WITH AVOCADO CREAM SAUCE

4 small (or 2 large) zucchini, ends trimmed and made into noodles with a julienne peeler or spiralizer
1 avocado
1/2 cucumber, chopped

juice of 1/2 a lemon
1 clove garlic
2 Tbs almond or coconut milk 8 leaves basil
salt & pepper

GARNISH
halved cherry tomatoes
additional basil leaves

Procedure

1. Place zucchini spirals in a large bowl.
2. In a food processor, combine the remaining ingredients and process until smooth.
3. Toss the zucchini with the avocado sauce until fully coated.
4. Garnish with cherry tomatoes and basil leaves, season with more salt & pepper to taste.

Preparation Time: 10 minutes
Total Time: 10 minutes

Source
Author: Unbound Wellness

DR. BUMP'S SNACKS RECIPES

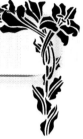

3 INGREDIENT HOMEMADE ALMOND CRACKERS

1 cup almond flour (not almond meal)

3 Tbs water

1 Tbs ground flaxseed

1/2 tsp fine sea salt

flaked sea salt (optional)

Procedure

1. Add almond flour, water, ground flaxseed, and sea salt into a medium sized bowl and stir together until the mixture turns into dough.

2. Place the dough on a piece of parchment paper. Cover it with a second piece of parchment. Pat it out with your hands and then use a rolling pin to roll out the dough. You'll want the dough to get pretty thin — about an 1/8 of inch thick. Try to form the dough into a rectangular shape. It's okay if it's not perfect.

3. Once the dough is rolled out, remove the top sheet of paper and sprinkle a bit of flaked sea salt over the dough. Use your hands to press the salt down to help it stick. This step is optional, but the flaked sea salt makes the crackers really pretty.

4. With the top sheet of parchment removed, use a pizza wheel or knife to cut the dough into small squares. I made mine about 1/2 -1 inch. If you want to get fancy you can use a tooth pick to create a little hole in the center of each cracker.

5. Move parchment paper to a baking sheet and bake the crackers for 20-25 minutes or until the crackers turn golden brown and crispy. The pieces on the outer edges will get brown faster than the center pieces. You can transfer those that are golden to a cooling rack and put the pan back in the oven to bake the remaining crackers.

6. Let the crackers cool completely, either on the baking sheet or on a cooling rack. Enjoy immediately after cooling. Place any leftover crackers in an airtight bag for later. You can store these in an air-tight

container or bag and keep them on the counter or pantry. They should last about 4-5 days.

Preparation Time: 10 minutes
Total Time: 30 minutes

Source
Author: Brittany Mullins

BAKED SWEET POTATO CHIPS

1 1/2 lbs sweet potatoes
1/3 cup olive oil
Salt

Procedure

1. Preheat the oven to 300 degrees F. Line several baking sheets with parchment paper and set aside. Use a mandolin slicer to cut the sweet potatoes into paper-thin rounds. (I set mine to the thinnest setting.) You can use a knife to do this, but it takes much longer.
2. Pile all the sweet potato rounds into a large bowl and pour the olive oil over the top. Gently toss to coat every piece with oil. Then lay the sweet potato rounds out on the baking sheets in a single layer.
3. Sprinkle the chips lightly withr Salt. Bake for 20-25 minutes until crisp and golden around the edges. Remove from the oven and cool for 5 minutes on the baking sheets. Then move the chips to a bowl, or plastic bag to store. If you happen to find a few chips with soft centers, pop them back in the oven for about 5 minutes.

Servings: 8

Preparation Time: 10 minutes
Cooking Time: 20 minutes
Total Time: 30 minutes

Recipe Tips
Sweet potato chips go from perfect to burnt very quickly. Start watching each batch at the 20 minute mark and remove them the moment they look 90% crispy. They will continue to crisp up as they cool.

Source
Author: Spicy Perspective

CAN'T STOP EATING 'EM CRISPY GREEN BEAN CHIPS

1 tsp each garlic powder and onion powder
5 lbs green beans (organic preferred)
1/3 cup oil (melted coconut oil preferred)
4 tsp salt
1 tsp each garlic powder and onion powder

Procedure

1. Place green beans in a large bowl. If using frozen green beans, simply allow them to thaw in a bowl (optional - see notes below). If using fresh beans, you will need to blanch them first.
2. Pour oil on top of beans. If using coconut oil, melt the oil first and work fast as the oils solidifies quickly if your room or beans are cold.
3. Sprinkle seasonings on top of coated beans and stir well.
4. Dry in dehydrator until crisp dry. This takes approximately 10 - 12 hours at 125 degrees, or 8 hours at 135 degrees, but occasionally longer. You could also bake in a low temperature oven.
5. Store in an airtight container.

Source
Author: a Whole New Mom

Author Notes
Leave Chips in Dehydrator: The chips need to be really really dry in order to be crispy. If you remove them from the dehydrator too soon, they will be really hard to chew.

Use Either Frozen or Thawed Beans: I have used both frozen and thawed beans. The oils solidifies quickly on them, but it does work.

DETOX FRIENDLY TRUFFLES

1/2 cup coconut oil
1/4 tsp salt
1/4 cup rice syrup
1 cup cacao powder

1/2 tsp vanilla
1/4 cup of almond butter
1/4 tsp cinnamon

Procedure

1. Melt coconut oil and transfer to bowl
2. Add salt, rice syrup, vanilla to oil and whisk
3. Add the rest of the ingredients and stir and stir and stir :)
4. Add the 'add in's' that you desire
   Couple tbsp. of cold water as needed to make the dough moldable
   Add any of the following AND you can roll the little balls that you make
   with the dough in these: walnuts, chia seeds, unsweetened coconut
5. Take a small amount in your hand and make small balls. If it's hard
   to work with, put dough in the refrigerator for a few minutes. Roll
   small balls in your coconut, walnuts, etc.
6. Put in the freezer when done. When solid you can then keep them
   in the refrigerator.

Source
Author: Dawn Bump

DETOX FRIENDLY VEGAN ALMOND BUTTER COOKIES

1 cup almond flour
1/2 tsp salt
1/4 tsp baking soda
1/2 cup of almond butter
1/4 cup rice syrup

2 Tbs warmed coconut oil or ghee
1 tsp vanilla extract
(I like to add a sprinkle of
cinnamon and/or cardamom for
flavor, but it is optional)

Procedure

1. Preheat the oven to 350 degrees
2. In small bowl combine almond flour, salt and baking soda
3. In a medium bowl mix almond butter, rice syrup, coconut oil (or ghee), and vanilla.
4. Blend dry ingredients into wet until combined.
5. Scoop dough in small balls onto parchment paper lined baking sheet
6. Use a fork to flatten in a criss-cross pattern (You can top cookies with unsweetened coconut or walnuts if desired)
7. Bake at 350 for 6 - 12 minutes until golden around the edges.

Source
Author: Dawn Bump

GUACAMOLE DEVILED EGGS

This recipe is not detox diet compliant

6 large eggs - hard boiled
1 medium haas avocado
2-3 tsp fresh lime juice
1 tsp red onion (minced)
1 Tbs minced jalapeno

1 Tbs fresh cilantro (chopped)
kosher salt and fresh ground pepper
(to taste)
1 Tbs diced tomato
pinch chili powder (for garnish)

Procedure

1. Peel the cooled hard boiled eggs.
2. Cut the eggs in half horizontally, and set the yolks aside.
3. In a bowl, mash the avocado and 2 whole egg yolks; discard the rest.
4. Mix in lime juice, red onion, jalapeño, cilantro, salt and pepper and adjust to taste. Gently fold in tomato.
5. Scoop heaping spoonfuls of the guacamole into the 12 halved eggs.
6. Sprinkle with a little chili powder for color and arrange on a platter.

Preparation Time: 30 minutes
Total Time: 30 minutes

Source
Author: Skinny Taste

LOW CARB CAULIFLOWER HUMMUS

3 cups cauliflower florets steamed

2 Tbs water

2 Tbs avocado or olive oil

1/2 tsp salt

3 whole roasted garlic cloves

1.5 Tbs Tahini paste

3 Tbs lemon juice

2 raw garlic cloves, crushed (in addition to above)

3 Tbs extra virgin olive oil

3/4 tsp kosher salt

smoked paprika and extra olive oil for serving

Procedure

1. Combine the steamed cauliflower, 2 Tbsp avocado or olive oil, 1/2 tsp kosher salt in a saute pan, simmer 5-10 minutes – or until softened and darkened in color
2. Put the cauliflower mixture into a magic bullet, blender, or food processor and blend. Add the tahini paste, roasted garlic, lemon juice, 2 raw garlic cloves, 3 Tbsp olive oil, and 3/4 tsp salt. Blend until mostly smooth. Taste and adjust seasoning as necessary
3. To serve, place the hummus in a bowl and drizzle with extra virgin olive oil and a sprinkle of paprika. Use celery sticks, raw radish chips, or other vegges to dip with.

Servings: 1

Source
Author: Mellissa Sevigny

NO-SUGAR ADDED CHIA SEED PUDDING

1/3 cup chia seeds
1 cup unsweetened vanilla almond milk dash of cinnamon and nutmeg or pumpkin pie spice
1/4 tsp vanilla 2/3 cup frozen fruit

Procedure

1. Place the chia seeds, almond milk, cinnamon, nutmeg or pumpkin pie spice in a jar or bowl.
2. Stir until well combined.
3. Stir in the frozen fruit. It may make your mixture seem like there are frozen clumps; it's okay.
4. Stir as best you can.
5. Place in the fridge and let the mixture sit for a couple hours, or ideally, over night.
6. After a couple hours or when you wake up, stir the pudding again so the fruit juices can spread some more.
7. Enjoy! Top with extra thawed fruit and some chopped nuts if you desire.
8. If you are unhappy with the texture you can blend it up in the blender.

Source
Author: Unknown

DR. BUMP'S SOUP RECIPES

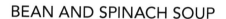

BEAN AND SPINACH SOUP

2 cups white kidney beans (cannellini) canned or home cooked
1-2 cups kidney or red beans, canned or home cooked
1 cup garbanzo beans (chickpeas) canned or home cooked
2-3 cups spinach or escarole. washed, drained, and chopped or 10 ounce frozen chopped spinach
4 cups vegetable broth
2 medium onions coarsely chopped
1 large clove garlic -- minced
1 tsp dried basil
1 Tbsp dried parsley
1 tsp dried oregano
Pepper to taste

Procedure

1. Combine all ingredients and simmer about 45 minutes, until inions are soft.

Servings: 6

Source
Author: LivClear recipes booklet

CABBAGE ROLL SOUP

1 lb ground beef
1 tsp sea salt
1/4 tsp black pepper
1 onion, diced
3-4 cloves garlic, minced
1 cup carrots, roughly chopped
1 cup cauliflower, riced

1 medium green cabbage, chopped
(about 4 cups)
5 cups beef broth
1 1/2 cup tomato sauce
Juice of half a lemon
2 tsp oregano
2 Tbs parsley, chopped

Procedure

1. Using a large, heavy cast iron pan or stock pot, brown the ground beef over medium heat. Lightly season and use a wooden spoon to crumble. Once browned, set aside and leave about 2 Tbsp of fat in the pan (or add avocado oil if needed).
2. Add the onion to the same pot and cook for 3-4 minutes or until lightly translucent. Add in the garlic, carrots, and cauliflower rice and cook for another 3-4 minutes to lightly soften. Stir in the cabbage and allow to wilt for 2 minutes
3. Add the beef back to the pot and stir in the broth, tomato sauce, lemon juice and oregano. Stir well and bring to a low simmer.
4. Allow to simmer for 30-35 minutes. The vegetables should be softened and the soup should lightly reduce.
5. Season the soup to taste and top with fresh parsley to serve.

Servings: 4

Preparation Time: 10 minutes
Cooking Time: 40 minutes
Total Time: 50 minutes

Source
Author: MICHELLE
Source: Unbound Wellness

CHICKEN POT PIE SOUP

2 Chicken breasts, large boneless skinless diced
3 Carrots (diced, 1 cup)
3 stalks Celery diced
5 cloves Garlic
1 Onion (diced, 1 cup)
1 Parsley, fresh leaves
1 lb white sweet potatoes diced
1 1/2 tsp Sage, dried
2 Tbs Thyme, fresh leaves

2 cups Chicken broth
1 Black pepper, freshly cracked
1 1/2 tsp Salt
Oils & Vinegars
2 Tbs Ghee or olive oil
Nuts & Seeds
1 cup Cashews
1 cup Coconut cream or milk, full-fat canned

Procedure

1. Soak cashews in warm water for at least 20 minutes drain off water
2. Meanwhile saute the celery, onion & carrots in olive oil or ghee on saute setting in instant pot until softened
3. Add garlic and stir for 30 seconds
4. Add diced chicken and saute until no longer pink
5. Add remaining ingredients except for coconut cream (add the softened cashews at this point)
6. Then pressure cook for 10 minutes on high
7. Let pressure release, and then stir in coconut cream until combined

Source
Author: unknown

Author Notes
You can also cook this recipe in a heavy pot, the only difference would be the cooking time, adjust to 45 minutes after everything has been added. Add in the coconut cream at the end and stir to combine

PALEO EGG ROLL SOUP

1 Tbs ghee, avocado oil, or olive oil
1 lb ground pastured pork
1 large onion, diced
32 oz (4 cups) chicken or beef broth
1/2 head cabbage, chopped
2 cups shredded carrots
1 tsp garlic powder

1 tsp onion powder
1 tsp sea salt
1 tsp ground ginger
2/3 cup coconut aminos
Optional: 2-3 tablespoons tapioca starch

Procedure

1. In your Instant Pot in saute mode brown the ground pork in the tablespoon of cooking fat with the diced onion; cook until no longer pink, cancel saute mode.
2. Add in the remaining ingredients cook under pressure for 25 minutes on high pressure then quick release the pressure
3. Remove lid and serve
4. If you want a thicker soup, remove 1/4 cup of broth from the soup and stir in 2-3 tablespoons of tapioca starch. Reintroduce the slurry and stir well, it will thicken over the next few minutes

Source
Author: predominantlypaleo.com/paleo-egg-roll-soup/

Printed in the United States
by Baker & Taylor Publisher Services